...and may just inspire the
that women have been
enjoying for decades."   —*Dish Magazine*

"Harvard Professor Dr. Abraham Morgentaler, founder of a Boston
clinic for male sexual and reproductive disorders, offers a glimpse
behind the examination-room door at the hopes and hang-ups of
his patients. His latest book, [*The Truth About Men and Sex*]
takes the measure of manhood in the age of Viagra, Internet porn,
and shifting gender roles."   —*Maclean's* (Canada)

"I can't remember the last time a piece of important medical history
made me gasp, drop my jaw, and then explode into disbelieving
laughter. But such was the effect of . . . Dr. Abraham Morgentaler's
new book, [*The Truth About Men and Sex*]."   —WBUR.org

"A tell-all exposé . . . [*The Truth About Men and Sex*] is a throw-
back that unfolds via the anecdotal weight of a seasoned doctor's
observations and his recollections of intimate details told to him
by his patients. Morgentaler expertly walks us through a host of
explanations for this scourge of denouement fictus. Indeed, [*The
Truth About Men and Sex*] unfolds like a present-day version of
the 1950s-era women's magazine self-help column Tell Me Doctor,
only here the patients are men. Thus we learn a great deal about
male biology."   —*Public Books*

"Morgentaler's experienced perspective comes across in his writing and will appeal to a wide audience. Eye opening and never
dull, this is a book both male and female readers interested in
medicine, sexuality, gender issues, and relationships will enjoy."
                                              —*Library Journal*

"An engaging, provocative, and fun book that moved me and also made me laugh. I will never think about men, sex, and relationships the same way again."

—Sanjiv Chopra, MD, professor of medicine at Harvard Medical School and author of *Live Better, Live Longer*

"Dr. Morgentaler takes us on a compelling journey into the minds of men and how they really feel about sex, love, and relationships. A great read for women who want to understand their lover's struggles and secret desires in the bedroom and beyond."

—Laura Berman, LCSW, PhD, author of *Loving Sex: The Book of Joy and Passion*

"Many novels and news stories describe 'hyper-sexed' men who care only about the pleasure sex gives to them, while others address the latest treatments for male sexual problems. But most men fit neither description. Most men can have sex, and have concerns about how well they satisfy their partners. For such men— and there are many of them—this book from a physician expert in men's sexual function has much valuable information. Clearly written, with compelling personal stories that make the material come alive."

—Anthony Komaroff, MD, professor of medicine at Harvard Medical School

"Dr. Morgentaler, a distinguished Harvard urologist, takes us into his consulting room and exposes the deep struggles and concerns that men have regarding their sexuality. Using humor and sensitivity, he reveals the interwoven physical and psychological concerns that are part and parcel of male sexual identity. [*The Truth About Men and Sex*] is a brave, bold, and extremely well-written book that teaches us about the complexity of the mind of man."

—Stanley E. Althof, PhD, executive director of the Center for Marital and Sexual Health of South Florida, emeritus professor at Case Western Reserve University School of Medicine

ALSO BY DR. ABRAHAM MORGENTALER

Testosterone for Life:
Recharge Your Vitality, Sex Drive,
Muscle Mass and Overall Health

The Viagra Myth:
The Surprising Impact on Love and Relationships

The Male Body:
A Physician's Guide to What Every Man
Should Know About His Sexual Health

THE TRUTH ABOUT MEN AND SEX

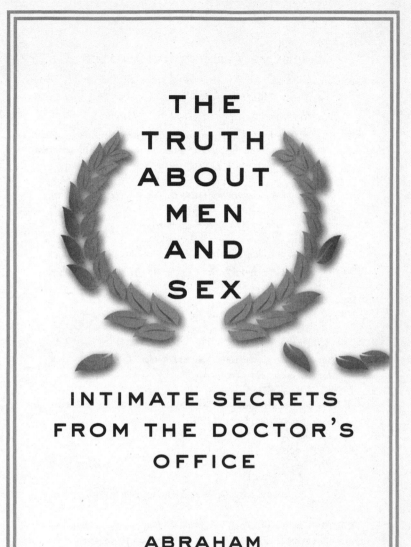

INTIMATE SECRETS FROM THE DOCTOR'S OFFICE

ABRAHAM MORGENTALER, MD

ST. MARTIN'S GRIFFIN NEW YORK

THE TRUTH ABOUT MEN AND SEX. Copyright © 2013 by Abraham Morgentaler. All rights reserved. Printed in the United States of America. For information, address St. Martin's Press, 175 Fifth Avenue, New York, N.Y. 10010.

www.stmartins.com

Designed by Meryl Sussman Levavi
Illustrations by Megan Rojas

The Library of Congress has cataloged the Henry Holt edition as follows:

Morgentaler, Abraham.
 Why men fake it : the totally unexpected truth about men and sex /
Abraham Morgentaler.
   p. cm.
 Includes bibliographical references and index.
 ISBN 978-0-8050-9424-4 (hardcover)
 ISBN 978-1-4299-4744-2 (e-book)
 1. Men—Sexual behavior.   2. Sex (Psychology)   3. Sexual health.
 4. Man-woman relationships.   I. Title.
 HQ28.M673 2013
 306.70811—dc23

                                    2012036217

ISBN 978-1-250-04260-6 (trade paperback)

St. Martin's Griffin books may be purchased for educational, business, or promotional use. For information on bulk purchases, please contact the Macmillan Corporate and Premium Sales Department at 1-800-221-7945, extension 5442, or write to specialmarkets@macmillan.com.

First published in hardcover under the title *Why Men Fake It*
by Henry Holt and Company, LLC

First St. Martin's Griffin Edition: March 2015

10 9 8 7 6 5 4 3 2

To Addy

CONTENTS

IV. THE MEASURE OF A MAN

A NOTE TO READERS

The stories presented in this book are based on actual cases during the author's twenty-five years of medical practice treating men with sexual and reproductive problems.

However, to preserve the privacy of his patients, names and details have been changed, and some cases presented are composite accounts, although those are also based on Doctor Morgentaler's actual clinical experiences.

The information in this book is not intended to replace the individualized advice of the reader's own physician or other medical professional. You should consult a medical professional in all matters relating to your health, especially if you have existing medical conditions, before deciding on any treatment, and before starting, stopping, or changing the dose of any medication.

Individual readers are solely responsible for their own health care decisions. The publisher does not accept responsibility for any adverse effects individuals may claim to experience, whether directly or indirectly, from the information contained in this book.

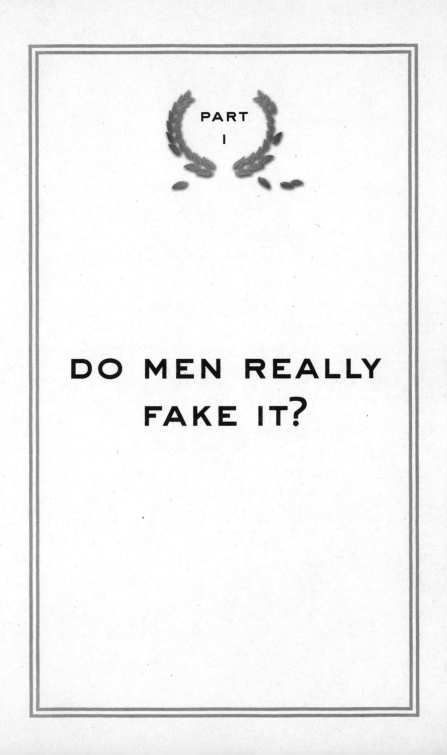

PART
I

DO MEN REALLY
FAKE IT?

I. INTRODUCTION

This is a book about the fascinating, rich, nuanced, and surprising world of men and sexuality. Over more than a quarter century of medical practice specializing in the treatment of men with sexual and reproductive conditions, I've been privileged to have been allowed entry into a secret world accessed by exceedingly few. Until I began this work as a young graduate of a high-powered training program in urology at Harvard Medical School, my views on male sexuality were informed primarily by what I saw on television or in movies, and what I saw among my friends and acquaintances. In other words, I knew nothing except stereotypes and bravado.

My education began immediately once my examination-room door closed and men dropped their guard in the hope that I could help them with their problems. I hadn't expected to hear the depth of feeling men expressed, and the complex ways that sex influenced the lives and relationships of my patients. My understanding of male sexuality was as superficial as the barely visible layer of ice atop a pond after the first overnight frost of the season. I wasn't alone in this, of course. Assaulted daily by sexual content in the media and on the Internet, it is easy to assume we are all experts in sexuality. Yet somehow we've managed to miss all the important stuff. Notably absent is any sense of what sex is like for men. What do men think about sex and relationships? What do they worry about, care about? What does a man need in order to feel manly? What do men *feel*?

If it is true that we only fully appreciate something when we no longer have it, and value it adequately only when it is regained, then in this age of Viagra, testosterone, and yes, even penile implants, there is now a remarkable opportunity to learn what sex means to a man. This book is my attempt to pull back the curtain and share whatever wisdom and experience accrues from a career of listening, treating, and observing. Honored by the trust and confidence of my patients and their partners, I offer their stories (with names and identifying details changed to preserve privacy) to challenge the tired, damaging male stereotypes, and to provide a modern perspective on men. There is no better way to explain what is true about men and sex than to share real stories from real men.

Comedians joke, "Why did God give men two brains but only enough blood to run one of them at a time?" Even in family-friendly newspaper comic strips we see men with eyes bulging out of their heads as a pretty woman walks by. The world of gender and sexuality has been turned upside down by events over the last forty years—women's liberation, the advent of the birth control pill, the high prevalence of women in the workforce, and the introduction of Viagra, to name just a few—yet these jokes about men and sex could have been lifted almost completely unchanged from the late 1960s and early 1970s when I was a teenager.

We live at a moment in history when we have more data about sex at our fingertips than at any time before, and yet we know so little about male sexuality. If we are so ignorant of basic information, how well can we hope to have a true and meaningful understanding of something as complex as the male psyche when it comes to sex?

It's not easy being a man these days, and certainly not a sexual man. Seismic changes in our social landscape have fractured the era of male dominance. As the father of two capable young women, I applaud the leveling of the gender playing field. Yet it is naive to assume there has not been a cost to this relatively sudden cultural change. There are now far fewer opportunities for men to feel powerful, and well, manly.

Recently, Mara and George—both thirty-two, with two young sons—came to see me in my office. George was a building contractor, Greek, a little stocky, with a round face, a solid-looking man. "Mara doesn't think we have sex enough," George said. "I start my days at five AM, I want to play with the kids when I get home, and then most days I collapse after dinner. Mara thinks it's strange that I'm too tired to have sex more than once or twice a week."

I looked toward Mara, pretty, slender, with dark, long hair. She looked very fit. "Doctor, I don't understand. I thought guys were supposed to always want sex. And before I had the kids, George *was* always ready. Now I want it, and he doesn't. Is it me? I worked hard to get rid of the baby fat from my pregnancy, but it doesn't seem to matter to him. I've asked him whether he's found someone else, and he says 'No,' but I just don't get it."

Alone with me during his examination, George took the opportunity to tell me more. "Doc, it's worse than you can imagine. Mara is sure I'm cheating. She's been snooping through all my stuff. I feel like I constantly have to reassure that we're okay, that I still find her sexy, that I still love her. It's a bad time for my business, and I'm stressed. Truthfully, some of the time we have sex, I'm doing it just to keep Mara happy." The idea that a man would have sex with a woman for her benefit rather than his own runs counter to the traditional story line about the selfish, egotistic sexual male seeking only his own gratification. Yet there is nothing unusual about George's story. Women have always had expectations from their men; now this expectation has shifted in new ways to the bedroom.

A young man in his midthirties without any problems with erections made an appointment to see me, in the hopes of receiving a prescription for Viagra. When I asked why he thought he needed it, he responded, "It's tough out there, Doc. The last woman I dated told me when she wanted sex, how she wanted it, and how many times she needed it. I'm just trying to keep up!"

It *is* tough out there for men. The world is changing rapidly and the misinformation that passes as conventional wisdom about male sexuality leads many men to have anxiety, low self-esteem, and conflict within relationships.

Let's get something straight about sex. Sex is how animals reproduce, from the smallest single-cell organism to insects, fish, reptiles, birds, and mammals. We tend to forget about the reproductive part because humans have been clever enough to find ways to separate sex from reproduction via various forms of contraception. What is important to understand is that the drive for sex is not a choice, nor a human invention. It is one of the most powerful drivers for all species on this planet. If tuna didn't have a powerful sex drive, there would be no tuna. If dogs didn't have a powerful sex drive, there would be no dogs. And if humans (male *and* female) didn't have a powerful sex drive, there would be no humans. This is a biological fact.

My perspectives on sexuality were influenced greatly by my initial choice of biology as a career. In my very first class as an undergraduate at Harvard College, the Nobel Prize laureate George Wald presented the big bang theory and described the subsequent primordial soup that eventually led to organic molecules and the beginnings of life. I was hooked. For three years as an undergraduate I worked in the reptile laboratory of the brilliant biologist David Crews, PhD (now at the University of Texas at Austin), studying the effects of testosterone on the sexual behavior of male lizards. Reptiles are extremely important in evolution because they represent the common ancestor of the "higher" animals, namely birds and mammals. It is the primitive reptilian portion of our brain that drives our sexual behavior, with input from higher centers in the cerebral cortex.

It makes perfect sense that the sexual centers in the human brain are deep, old in evolutionary terms, and anatomically distinct from the "thinking" part of our brain, namely the cerebral cortex, because sex has very little to do with thinking. Indeed, lust, libido, sex drive—whatever one wishes to call it—seems to be almost a form of madness. It is irrational, primal. In the throes of lust, women and men behave differently than in every other sphere of our lives. Individuals who are germophobic and who wouldn't dare to touch a doorknob without first wiping it down with a cloth will, when sexually excited, throw themselves into skin-on-skin, sweat-on-sweat, full-body contact with another person, exchanging body fluids along the way. Powerful men and women who experience rage at any perceived disrespect at work engage happily in sex play in which they are subdued, dominated, demeaned. Sex is a break in the normal fabric of our lives. One can no more reasonably separate sexual desire from normal men and women than one can separate wetness from water.

Despite our sexual nature, it is unacceptable to be sexual whenever the urge arises. All human societies have found ways to bind our sexuality by rules, norms, culture. It is endlessly fascinating to me how we manage to incorporate the "madness" of our sexuality within the framework of a rational life in which we aspire to be honorable and productive. One of the consequences of the inevitable tension between primitive urges and civilized behavior has been to make sexuality into a big secret, something not practiced in public, and not spoken about.

I would argue that a key component of the women's movement and the rise of feminism was the way that women educated themselves about their bodies and their sexuality. A landmark event in the 1970s was the publication of *Our Bodies, Ourselves*, a book with graphic illustrations that could be found on almost every woman's college bookshelf; the book encouraged women to take a mirror and examine their genitalia, find their clitoris, and to experiment with masturbation so that they could experience orgasms more easily. It explained anatomy, menstruation, birth control, the whole works.

There has never been a similar book for men, at least not one that gained any national attention. A book that explained, discussed, and *normalized* male sexual behavior. Perhaps this book can start the conversation. Certainly there is a need for such a dialogue, for the benefit of women as well as men.

What will emerge from the stories in this book is that men are complex, thoughtful, and eager to be a valued and respected partner. It will be surprising to many to learn that man's sense of his own masculinity is intimately related to his ability to regard himself as a sexual provider.

There are other challenges to overcome in the realm of male sexuality besides ignorance, particularly physical ones. The medical world was stunned when results of the Massachusetts Male Aging Study in 1994 revealed that 52 percent of relatively healthy men between the ages of forty and seventy years reported some degree of impotence. So many men! We never knew.

Premature ejaculation affects as many as 20 percent of young men and nearly an equal number of older men. It is difficult to feel great about oneself as a lover when sex ends almost as soon as it begins. And new data shows that one-third of men over the age of forty-five have low levels of testosterone, which can cause poor erections, low sex drive, and difficulty achieving an orgasm.

By providing a behind-the-closed-door perspective on men, sex, and relationships, I hope that we will move out of the darkness and toward a more realistic, and kinder, view of what men are all about and how their minds work. Female readers may be happy to learn there *are* good men out there. And male readers may take comfort from realizing that they are not alone. The truth is that men are so much more interesting and complex than we would ever have believed.

2. THE MAN WHO
FAKED HIS ORGASMS

The secret of success is sincerity. Once you can fake that you've got it made.

—JEAN GIRAUDOUX (1882–1944), French novelist

One of the great misconceptions of male sexuality is that men are only concerned with their own orgasm. The classic stereotype is the guy who rolls over and falls asleep once he's climaxed, unaware or uncaring that his partner might still need a wee bit of stimulation in order to be satisfied herself.

This stereotype is inaccurate. Men feel awful if they believe they have sexually disappointed their partner. Does this mean that the "slam, bam, thank you, ma'am" attitude of men is total fiction? Of course not. Some men, and some men under certain circumstances (e.g., hookups where there is no emotional connection), really do not care about pleasing their partners. But in my practice, I have yet to meet a man who did not wish to be regarded as a knowledgeable, capable lover.

Sal, a forty-two-year-old muscular construction worker, cried in my office upon sharing with me that after twenty-one years of marriage his wife had just told him that she'd never had an orgasm with him during sex. "All this time I thought everything was okay, that I was giving her pleasure." He dabbed at his eyes with the tissue I handed him. "I never knew. I'm nothing now. I can't even call myself a man!" he exclaimed through his tears, disgusted with himself.

Sal had no idea whether his wife was even able to experience an orgasm at all. Indeed, various studies have reported that between 15 and 25 percent of women in the United States are anorgasmic, that is, unable to achieve an orgasm. And many women who do have orgasms find it impossible to get there via intercourse, requiring direct manual stimulation of their clitoris. Sal was down on himself for not "satisfying" his wife, without knowing whether or not it said something about him as a man.

Of course, a woman's degree of satisfaction may be difficult to read for a man. One would assume that if she had multiple screaming orgasms, a man could take comfort in a job well done. Not necessarily. Joseph was a thirty-eight-year-old, recently divorced man in a new relationship. "Fiona was much more experienced than me. One day after sex she held up three fingers to me, and I asked, 'Three what?' and she told me she'd just had three orgasms. That sounded pretty good to me, but I wasn't really sure. I'd never been with a woman who could have multiple orgasms. In magazines, though, I'd read that some women can have a dozen orgasms in a row just by fantasizing or by squeezing their legs together. So even though three orgasms *sounded* good to me, I worried that maybe Fiona had expected more from me. Later, when I asked if it was good or bad that she'd had three O's, she kicked me so hard in the shin that I still had the welt two weeks later!"

Men find the female orgasm mysterious since it seems so much more complex and variable than their own, which we think of as automatic. Moreover, the female orgasm isn't accompanied by an ejaculation to make things obvious. Yet the male orgasm has its own share of complexity.

David, whom I introduced earlier, was a nice-looking engineer, twenty-eight years old, with wavy, dark brown hair and dark, deep-set eyes. He wore a baseball cap turned backward. Black

T-shirt over a trim torso, blue jeans ripped over both thighs, and slightly distressed leather loafers completed an image that said, "I am one hip dude." On the intake questionnaire David had encapsulated the reason for his visit in a single word: *ejaculation*.

"How can I help you?" I asked, once we were seated after introductions. Based on what he had written on his intake form, I expected David to tell me that he ejaculated too quickly, by far the most common sexual complaint among young men. However, his problem was more unusual.

"I can't have an orgasm during sex," he answered. "It's no problem when I'm by myself," he continued. "It's just an issue when I'm with a woman."

"Tell me about it," I said.

"It's been this way my whole life. I've had my share of girlfriends, and I've just never been able to come during sex. Well"—he corrected himself—"maybe once or twice, but not in quite a few years. It's never been a real problem, though. As a matter of fact, because I could keep going and going, a lot of the girls I dated thought I was a stud. I've had girls tell me that most guys came before they had time to get off themselves, but with me they didn't need to worry about it because I lasted so long. That made me feel good. For years I thought I had a special gift because I didn't come during sex."

"So what brings you to see me now?"

"It's because of Sarah." He paused. "We've been dating for a few months, and we're really into each other. Sex has been a problem, though. I started off doing my usual thing, but after the second or third time we hooked up, she told me she thought it was weird that I didn't come. I told her it was probably just because I was nervous. It bothered her that she couldn't get me off, even though I told her I was fine. Sarah is pretty hot, and she said she'd never been with a guy who didn't come during sex. I think it made her worry that I'm not that into her, or that she doesn't know how to do it right for me.

"She is persistent, though." He smiled wryly. "One night I could tell she was on a mission to make me come. She tried everything, and we kept going until I was raw. I was sore the whole day afterward." David broke eye contact with me and turned his gaze downward. That's when he confessed his unusual practice. "I faked an orgasm that night. And now I fake it whenever we have sex.

"I don't like doing it, but it works for now. Sarah seems to enjoy sex more, and the relationship is going great otherwise."

"How do you fake it?"

"When I figure it's time, I do the whole thing. I groan and tense up for a while and then relax." David described this as if it were the most natural thing any man might do.

I was trying to take it all in, but I was still stuck on something. "Tell me again, *why* do you fake your orgasms with Sarah?" I asked.

"Sarah is a beautiful woman, but I could tell she was feeling bad about herself because I couldn't come. Less feminine, less sexy. She was getting frustrated with sex, even though she always came with me. Faking my orgasm seemed like an easy, harmless way to solve the problem. And it worked. Sarah is much happier now, and the sex is great."

"It sounds as if you've come upon an ingenious solution. How can I help?"

"Sarah is under the impression that I didn't come at the beginning because I was nervous and needed time to get comfortable with her. She thinks my ability to have an orgasm more quickly now is a sign that we're doing better together. It's okay for right now, but I'm afraid Sarah will figure it out eventually." David inhaled deeply and gathered himself. "This is the most serious relationship I've ever been in. Sarah might even be 'the one,' if you know what I mean. She's big into honesty, though, and if she found out I was faking it, I don't think we'd survive it. She'd be too hurt. And I can just imagine her calling me a faker, an imposter. I need you to help me start having orgasms during sex."

It was Barry, a patient of mine, who convinced me that it may not be all that rare for a man to fake an orgasm. When I asked him if he'd ever done it, he replied, "No. Of course not—why would I? But I dated a girl once who I thought was a little crazy. Every time we had sex, she would stop me on my way to the bathroom and inspect the condom before I pulled it off, checking the end of it. It seemed strange to me, but I figured she was nervous about getting pregnant and was checking for a leak. So one day I asked her why she did that. She said, 'I'm checking to make sure you really came.' What a nut! How could a man ever fake an orgasm?" he wondered aloud.

Too Slow, Too Quick

Whenever I've shared David's story I've heard two fairly uniform responses. Women say, "That's impossible! There's no way a guy could fake it!" usually followed by, "And if a guy were crazy enough to *try* to fake it with me, I'd know for sure." The response from men tends to be a more quizzical: "Why would a man need to fake it?"

Indeed, most readers would find it difficult to imagine that a healthy young man like David would be unable to have an orgasm during sex. Many men have experienced sex as a lifelong pitched battle to stave off a too-quick orgasm. In fact, in order to prolong the sexual encounter, and to increase the likelihood that the woman will also have time to reach a climax, men have hit upon some curious strategies to *avoid* orgasm.

"Think about death" is a classic chestnut passed on to inexperienced men to help them avoid the embarrassment of premature ejaculation. Another is "Imagine you're having sex with your mother," a disturbing idea with the potential to precipitate a Freudian crisis. Some men have even told me they've tried to delay ejaculation by causing themselves pain during sex, attempting to undercut the irrepressible delicious feelings with noxious sensations—bending their toes against the bedpost or biting their forearms, sometimes breaking the skin. Ouch! Men do what they can to delay ejaculation because they feel inadequate when it happens too quickly; they fear they have disappointed their partner. Although some men with premature ejaculation might wish upon a magic lantern that they could trade their rapid ejaculation for no ejaculation at all in order to be a more successful lover, David's story illustrates that this poses its own set of challenges.

Strange as it may seem, David's difficulty achieving an orgasm (a condition called delayed, or retarded, ejaculation) can be caused by a number of medical conditions. It can result from side effects of certain medications. Sometimes the problem is due to a physical interaction between man and partner that is insufficiently exciting or even unpleasant ("she looks so bored"). And sometimes it can be psychological.

Timing

In sex, as in comedy, timing is key. One doesn't think about it much, but timing during sex is more complicated than it might appear. Imagine that both partners are able to have an orgasm within three seconds after beginning sexual activity. Mission accomplished, no effort or sweat required. Would that be a good experience?

In Woody Allen's futuristic movie *Sleeper* (1973), the women are all "frigid," that is, unable to climax, and all the men are impotent, "except those with Italian ancestors," deadpans Diane Keaton's character. The solution to this sexual impasse is a machine called the Orgasmatron, which provides a nearly instantaneous orgasmic experience for couples who enter the tiny cylinder. When Allen's character is chased by the police, he hides alone in the Orgasmatron and closes the door behind him, activating the machine. Moments later the doors open and the police escort him away, hair mussed, a silly grin on his face.

I don't think we're at risk of an Orgasmatron replacing sex, even if it were available today. The orgasm may be the payoff, but the buildup, the arousal, the crescendo toward a wonderful climax, is indisputably part of the pleasure of sex. And all of this takes time. For most men and women, an instantaneous orgasm without any additional activity would be a major disappointment. Sex is one of those activities where the journey is definitely as important as reaching the destination. This is a big part of the disappointment when a man ejaculates too rapidly.

David's story raises questions about the opposite circumstance: What if men and women had the capability to have sex indefinitely without orgasm? When would sex end? Although the idea of an endless night of sex sounds great in concept, there are practical issues ready to burst that bubble, like chafing. And sometimes life needs to go on, whether it's being ready for work in the morning or just getting enough sleep in order to be functional the next day.

A friend of mine once shared with me over drinks how excited he was about a new relationship. He and his new girlfriend were having sex "all night long." When I met up with him again a couple of weeks later he had dark bags under his eyes and looked haggard.

"You look exhausted," I told him.

"I am," he replied. "This woman I'm dating is a freak! She wants to have sex every night, for hours. I'm falling asleep at work, and I can't get anything done. I've got to break up with her—she's killing me!"

There is a downside to overly long sex, just as there is for sex that is too brief.

So how much time is enough? One of the challenges of sex is to be able to time it so that both individuals are satisfied. Usually it is the man who controls how long sex lasts, since once he comes the game is over, at least for a while. Yet indirectly, it is the woman who usually determines the duration of intercourse, since most women require more stimulation than men to climax, and the man will do what he can to defer his own orgasm until the woman comes. This unspoken "rule" of sex was cleverly captured by the title of the popular relationship book *She Comes First* by Ian Kerner. However, if the woman is among the 15 to 25 percent who cannot achieve an orgasm during sex at all, how long should a man continue sex play?

"Some nights I can tell it's just not going to happen for me," one woman explained to me. "It's not a big deal. But guys are so goal-oriented. With my last boyfriend, I had to fake an orgasm if I didn't think I was going to come, or else he'd be rubbing on me till tomorrow. Once he thought I'd had an orgasm, real or faked, he felt that he'd done a good job, and he'd let himself come too. And then we could both get some sleep."

David's practice of faking an orgasm turns this story on its head. So let's get to a critical question. Can a man really fake an orgasm?

Can a Man Really Fake It?

When David told me he faked his orgasms with Sarah, I immediately thought of the classic movie *When Harry Met Sally* (1989), in which the title characters, played by Billy Crystal and Meg Ryan, are in a deli discussing his love life. When Sally suggests that Harry's girlfriend is probably faking her orgasms with him, he says that would be impossible, because he would know if she were faking it. At which point Sally begins simulating a full-throated orgasm right there in the middle of the restaurant to prove how easy it is to fake it, building up to a crescendo of moans and groans, climaxing with "Yes! Yes!" When she's done, a woman at a nearby table tells the waiter, "I'll have whatever she's having."

We're familiar with the idea that a woman can fake an orgasm. It's an act, a performance, designed to make the man feel okay about himself, and to bring the activity to what feels like a satisfactory conclusion. But can a man fake it? The female response, "I would know instantly if a man tried to fake it with me," sounds suspiciously like Harry's in the movie.

When I pointed out this similarity to a female colleague, her response was "Oh no, it's different." And then, with a triumphal flourish, finger raised in the air like a prosecutor summing up a criminal case on television, she exclaimed, "With a man, there is evidence!"

Okay. Is that the extent of the argument? If there were no "evidence," that is, no semen, would a woman be able to tell if a man faked an orgasm? This raises a series of questions. Does fluid always come out when a man has an orgasm? Can he withhold it? What about if a man has had a vasectomy—is there still fluid that comes out? Before we can explore *why* David faked it, it is necessary to understand some of the incredible details regarding the biology of the male sexual response.

What Is Sex?

A visitor from another planet who landed in any grocery store checkout aisle in the United States and perused our magazines (assuming her advanced intellect allowed her to instantly understand English) might be excused for believing that earthlings do not reproduce via sex. If our visitor picked up a magazine like *Cosmopolitan*, she might read a dozen articles about sex (e.g., "Seven Amazing Sex Positions" or "Learn About His G-Spot"), with not a single word mentioned about pregnancy. Unless a person is actively interested in achieving a pregnancy, or preventing one, sexual thoughts are devoid of any reproductive content.

Sex has become an end in itself. There's nothing wrong with this, but it is useful to recognize the reproductive origins of sex if we are to understand our sexuality.

For the last twenty years I have taught a medical school class, lecturing to second-year students on the male contribution to fertility. For my first class, we review how sperm are made, how they mature, and how they are transported along the tubes within the body from the testicles* and eventually out the urethra. This first

---

* A point of terminology. There are two medical words that are interchangeable for a man's seat of power: *testicles* and *testes*, pronounced "test-ease" (the singular is *testis*, pronounced "tess-tis").

class is about the sperm "factory" and the transport pathways. My second class is about sex.

I begin with the statement "All animals have sex" and present a series of slides showing a variety of animals in the midst of sexual activity. "One-celled organisms do it," I explain, and show a cytoplasmic bridge between two microorganisms. "Insects do it," and a picture of mating flies appears. I continue with images of turtles, birds, and other creatures, all in the midst of having sex.

When an image of a mud-covered male hog mounting a female comes on the screen, I say, "I wonder if this male is worried about his body odor." The students snicker. And when a huge bison appears, mounting a female, I ask, "Is this male thinking about whether he is now supposed to call her tomorrow, or if this means they are now in a committed relationship?" The students laugh, because it seems so silly to think of these animals pondering relationship issues or being self-aware. Finally, I show my last slide, saying, "When it comes to sex, humans are different." An image then appears from the television show *Seinfeld* with the neurotic character George in bed with his girlfriend.

Thanks to human inventiveness, we have devised contraceptive methods that allow us to separate sex from reproduction. In developed countries fewer than 1 percent of all human sexual encounters result in a live birth, placing humans among the most reproductively inefficient species. Any animal in the wild with such a low fertility rate would quickly find itself on the endangered species list. For humans, though, this is the entire intent. Most of the time we want sex to be about nothing other than sex. For humans, sex can be regarded as a social event, arguably the most intense of our social interactions. Men and women may remember details of sexual encounters for years, even decades— the buildup, the flirting, the excitement, the minutiae of the act itself. We view sex among animals as natural, and instinctive, whereas for us it is an event, filled with conscious (and self-conscious) thoughts. Human sex is so much more than a biological imperative leading to a reproductively promising climax. We think, we choose, we hope, we worry, we wonder, we enjoy, we judge. How we feel about ourselves in sexual terms influences our over-all self-esteem. For men and women, sex is more than just a way to make a baby.

Orgasm and Ejaculation

From a reproductive perspective, the male contribution to sex and reproduction is straightforward. The man's penis becomes engorged with blood until it is firm enough to penetrate the vagina, and soon afterward sticky fluid is released, called semen or semi-nal fluid, which contains the sperm. That's it. The rest is up to the woman.

Not so fast. The details that lead up to this "simple" story are complex and fantastic. In chapter 6 I will describe in detail how erections work, but for the moment I want to focus on the release of semen, since this is a key to the puzzle of whether David could really fake his orgasms without Sarah knowing. First, a terminol-ogy quiz.

What is the difference between orgasm and ejaculation? This question seems easy enough, right? These are words everyone is familiar with. Do they have the same meaning? If not, how are they different? Don't feel bad if you don't know the difference. Every year I ask my second-year Harvard Medical students this question, and I'm still waiting for someone to answer it correctly.

Ejaculation and orgasm are two distinct biological events for men. The confusion arises because we use the terms for these events interchangeably. Under normal circumstances, if a man says "I ejaculated" or "I had an orgasm," it means the same to us, because both took place together. Here's a hint to teasing apart the differ-ent meanings: Can a woman have an orgasm? Of course. Can a woman ejaculate? Hmm. That's harder to answer, isn't it?

Orgasm is the full-body experience of reaching that magic point of release. The fireworks, if you will. *Climax* is merely a syn-onym for *orgasm*. Ejaculation, however, is the expulsion of the

sexual fluid. Orgasm and ejaculation normally occur simultane-
ously in men (which is why we tend to think of *orgasm* and *ejaculation* as interchangeable terms); however, there are a number of
circumstances in which they do not.

Do Women Ejaculate?

The idea that a faked orgasm is easier to detect in a man than a
woman based on the argument that "with a man there is evidence!"
suggests a major distinction in sexual function between the sexes.
However, it's not so simple. It turns out that some women do indeed
ejaculate. Many of these women are horribly ashamed of themselves because they and their doctors have assumed they were
leaking urine. This can also occur, but usually with women who
already have known problems with urine leakage, and is not necessarily associated with orgasm. Women who ejaculate release one
or several bursts of fluid from glands near the vaginal opening in a
pulsatile fashion similar to a man's ejaculation.

Not only do some women ejaculate like men, but the fluid
squirted out is biochemically similar to male semen and comes
from glands lining the urethra that are essentially a female equivalent of the male prostate. The major difference in the fluid is that
it doesn't contain sperm. Thus, whereas sexual experts once
asserted that both men and women can have an orgasm, but only
men ejaculate, it turns out this is just one more thing that men
cannot claim for themselves alone.

Where Did the Semen Go?

For David to be a successful faker-of-orgasms, he had to have
some way to handle the "evidence" for Sarah. Is it possible for a
man like David to have an orgasm without any fluid coming out?

Ejaculation in men is a key component of human reproduction. With orgasm, the man releases 1.5 to 5 cubic centimeters (for
reference, a teaspoon is 5 cc) of semen, which is a mixture of com-

ponents from three sources, combined at the critical moment of climax. About two-thirds of the fluid is produced by the seminal vesicles, a paired set of glands that lie just behind the prostate. For centuries, the seminal vesicles were believed to be a reservoir for sperm, but this is incorrect. The seminal vesicles produce fluid that is beneficial for the delicate sperm, with an alkaline pH and the sugar fructose, which serves as the primary energy source for sperm movement once they are ejaculated.

Most of the remaining fluid comes from the prostate, and a small portion, 5 to 10 percent, comes from the testicles, including the sperm. Thus, when a man has a vasectomy, he only loses the small amount that comes from the testicles. Most men don't even notice a difference in the amount of fluid after vasectomy, contrary to the common myth that vasectomy results in a dry ejaculation.

During the first moment of ejaculation, all three fluids are deposited into the urethra as it passes through the central part of the prostate. Powerful muscular contractions around the prostate and at the base of the penis forcibly and rhythmically expel the semen out the tip of the penis. To ensure that the fluid doesn't go backward into the bladder, the sphincter muscle at the junction of the bladder and prostate closes just before ejaculation. As men age, the expulsive forces are reduced and the semen comes out more slowly, oozing rather than spurting.

Normally, ejaculation is part of the orgasm experience, but not always. Sam was a sixty-two-year-old Ukrainian man who had undergone surgery for prostate cancer, an operation called radical prostatectomy. During the operation, the prostate and seminal vesicles are both removed in their entirety, and the tube carrying sperm from the testicles, called the vas deferens, is disconnected from the prostate. Thus everything that contributed fluid to the ejaculation is gone.

One of the common problems encountered by men who undergo this kind of surgery is poor erections, and this was what Sam wanted me to help him with. There were a number of options for Sam, but I also needed to learn more about his sexual functioning.

"Sam, how is your sex drive?" I asked.

"Strong!" he said with a smile.

"Can you have an orgasm?"

"What a question! Of course! But no fluid comes out. It feels the same, though, and I have the same throbbing sensation in my penis and behind my scrotum. Very satisfying, and an additional benefit is, no mess!"

For many men, however, the loss of semen can be quite disconcerting. One class of medication, called alpha blockers, can cause a severe reduction in the amount of semen that comes out with ejaculation, sometimes eliminating it completely. Alpha blockers are often prescribed for men with frequent or slow urination. As one patient, Brock, described it, "I was totally freaked out when I had sex and nothing came out of me. I didn't know what to think. Did I have cancer? Was there something wrong with my equipment? There were a couple of awful nights there when I didn't want to have sex. I was ticked off at my doctor that he didn't tell me this could happen from the medication."

There can be other medical reasons why a man might have an orgasm without ejaculation. In some men with diabetes or neurologic conditions, the urinary sphincter does not close properly at the beginning of orgasm, allowing the semen to seep into the bladder instead of coming out the tip of the penis, a condition called retrograde ejaculation. The sperm come out with the urine the next time the man urinates. Also, some operations can compromise the nerves controlling the ejaculatory process, leading to the same dry orgasm that Sam experienced.

With David, two main issues come to mind. The first is why he couldn't have an orgasm during sex, and the second is why and how he faked it.

"David, do you think Sarah can tell that you're faking?" I asked.

"I don't think so," he replied. "She seems pretty happy about our sex life. We're pretty active, and she gives me the impression she enjoys herself. If she knows, she's not saying anything."

"What about the fluid? Doesn't she notice that there's no semen?"

David shrugged. "I don't know. When we started seeing each other I used a condom, and I just made sure she didn't have a chance to check me out before I flushed it down the toilet. When we decided to be exclusive we both got tested and I stopped using condoms when our tests came back okay."

"You don't think Sarah notices there's no semen now that you don't use a condom?"

"Sarah gets pretty wet," he answered. "It seems to me there's already plenty of fluid, and it would be hard for her to tell."

There you have it. If the man does a good job hiding the absence of semen, there's really no reason a man can't fake an orgasm as well as a woman.

Creatures of Habit

David's underlying problem that led him to fake his orgasms was that he was unable to climax during intercourse. What could explain David's difficulty if it wasn't due to a medical condition?

Although the reflex to ejaculate is wired into our brains at the most primitive level, like all other higher animals, humans do have the ability to modify or influence this response. In fact, we can often train our bodies to do something different from what they seem inclined to do. Ramon's case is a good example. Ramon was a twenty-nine-year-old auto body detailer, originally from Puerto Rico, who owned his own shop. He was referred to me for infertility. He walked in with a bit of a swagger. His hair was slicked back, and he wore a pencil-thin beard that outlined the contours of his jaw. He was trim and wore a tight T-shirt and jeans. Ramon informed me that he and his wife, Suzy, had been unable to achieve a pregnancy for more than a year. A semen analysis had shown reduced numbers of sperm.

I reviewed Ramon's medical history, asking about medications, prior surgery, injuries to the genital region, and his use of alcohol, tobacco, and recreational drugs. There was nothing particularly notable that might contribute to his infertility. When I was done with my standard questions, I asked, "Is there anything else I should know?"

He fidgeted a bit. "Sex with Suzy . . ." His voice drifted off, and he made a face suggesting awkwardness with the conversation.

"Are you having trouble with erections?" I guessed. This is a frequent problem for men who feel the pressure to have sex "on command" when the timing is right, especially if there is any indication that the man may be contributing to the infertility.

"No." He seemed surprised and a bit offended. "My erections are okay. I just don't come inside."

It turned out that Ramon was incapable of ejaculating when his penis was inside the vagina. In the seven years that Ramon and Suzy had been together, he had never ejaculated inside her. Until recently, the couple had wanted to *avoid* a pregnancy, and the form of contraception they used is the oldest one in the book, called coitus interruptus ("interrupted sex"). When Ramon felt he was about to ejaculate he would pull his penis out of Suzy's vagina and ejaculate outside of her.

Once Ramon and Suzy decided to have children, however, Ramon found himself unable to shift gears. He told me proudly that he had begun being sexually active with girls at age fifteen and had never used a condom. Pulling out was his modus operandi, and this was how he had avoided any pregnancies in the past, with Suzy or with previous partners. Ramon had trained his body and took satisfaction in his ability to control himself in this way. Now that he and Suzy wanted children together, though, he found himself unable to change.

Ramon and I discussed different strategies to help him ejaculate intravaginally (within the vagina), but frankly, he wasn't interested. He and Suzy eventually had three children, all conceived by intrauterine insemination, in which Ramon produced a semen sample in a sterile cup, which was then processed, and the concentrated sperm sample was then inserted via a tiny straw into Suzy's uterus when she was ready to ovulate.

This would seem to be an easy problem to solve. After all, generations of men have had the opposite experience, namely trying to pull out just before climax, only to miss the timing by a beat or two, resulting in an unwanted pregnancy or at least a big scare. I'm sure if Ramon's friends were to hear his story, they would say to him, "Dude, just let it happen." Yet a lifetime of ejaculatory training, one could even call it discipline, is not so simple to undo and can make it difficult for a man to ejaculate "normally" during intercourse. It's worth mentioning that there was nothing wrong with the way Ramon and Suzy had sex. It's just that coitus interruptus is not a great way to get your wife pregnant.

Orgasm as Weakness?

There can be psychological reasons why a man may find himself unable to come during sex. Sylvester was a forty-two-year-old referred to me by his psychologist. Sylvester was handsome, trim, and muscular. He had never married and had no children. He worked as a consultant for a major business firm and traveled around the country to help improve efficiency and profits for struggling medium-to-large companies. "I find their weak spots and turn them into strengths," he explained.

"I don't come during sex," Sylvester said. "I never have. I'm single, and I meet a lot of women during my travels. I enjoy sex a lot—don't get me wrong. But I can keep going and going all night and never have an orgasm with a woman. I'm convinced it's psychological, but I figured I'd see you to make sure it wasn't something physical."

"Are you able to have an orgasm on your own?"

"Oh sure. That's no problem at all."

"Why do you believe it's psychological?"

Sylvester sighed and shifted in his seat. "My mother raised me in a small town in Alabama, together with three older sisters, who babied me. I never knew my father. When I reached a certain age I couldn't stand that environment anymore."

"I don't notice a southern accent," I commented.

"I took diction classes to lose the accent during my first semester at college. I thought it made me sound less sophisticated. Anyway, my shrink and I agree that my problem comes from being raised in a family of women."

"I don't understand."

"I refuse to let a woman see me as weak. Once, in college, I did come during sex with a girl. It was awful. She stroked my face, and I thought I just might as well die and get it over with right there. I grabbed my clothes and ran out of the room."

"Because she stroked your face?"

"You got it."

Sylvester was determined to not have any *weak spots*, to use his consulting terminology. For him, losing control during an orgasm was something he desperately wanted to avoid, and he had successfully managed to do so since that first and only episode.

Sylvester failed to see the beauty of how sex can lead to intimacy—shared moments of literal nakedness when our unmasked nature shows up. We learn to cover ourselves with so much armor every day, and over years and years it builds up, closing us off from shared experiences, shared lives. For those who are open to it, the intimacy of sex can strip away those layers. Yet the closeness and tenderness that Sylvester's college girlfriend may have felt for him at that moment of "weakness" was anathema to him, intolerable. Sylvester explained, "Consciously or unconsciously, I made a decision to never 'give it up' to a woman."

I examined Sylvester, and we spoke a bit more. I agreed there was no evidence for a physical problem, and that his condition was likely to be psychological, as he had already concluded. He seemed satisfied with this assessment. We stood up, shook hands, and he started toward the door.

"One last thing before you go," I said. Sylvester turned to face me. "After all these years, what made you decide to address this issue now?"

"My mother died last year. I don't need to prove anything to her anymore." He smiled with unnatural calm and strutted out the door.

For Sylvester, like Ramon, the failure to have an orgasm during sex was something he had trained himself to do, although for different reasons. It is fascinating how individuals can respond so differently to the same sexual event, such as an orgasm during intercourse, ranging from satisfaction ("Mmm") to ecstasy ("Wow!") to relief ("Finally!") to revulsion (e.g., Sylvester's reaction) to fear (e.g., of pregnancy) to self-reproach ("Ugh! I came too quickly!"). Sex for humans is complex, and men bring to it their own sets of personal histories and psychologies.

Helping David

As we've seen, there can be any number of reasons why a man may have difficulty achieving an orgasm during sex. Medical conditions, certain kinds of surgery, and side effects of medications can be trouble. Probably the most common cause is the antidepressant class of medications called selective serotonin reuptake inhibitors (SSRIs), which includes Prozac, Paxil, and Zoloft. Hormonal issues, specifically low levels of testosterone, can also make it difficult to achieve an orgasm. Men on SSRIs or with low testosterone describe a feeling where they may be very turned on during sex but can't quite get to the magical point of release. Aging can also be an issue, as it can cause reduced sensation and a requirement for more stimulation.

It can also be psychological, as demonstrated by Sylvester, when the subconscious develops reasons to *avoid* orgasm which overcome the natural biological urge *to have* an orgasm. I have seen this response in men with a fear of having children, even when using a condom, and in men whose strict religious training against the sins of premarital sex persisted into their marriages.

Occasionally, an otherwise wonderful partner can rub a man the wrong way. I've seen men who were bothered by the woman's scent ("Reminded me of my grandmother") or who complained that their partner was too rough. Other men have told me their partner acted disinterested in sex or made them feel guilty or intimidated ("She's had a lot of partners. I wasn't sure I would match up with what she was used to").

Finally, there are everyday practical considerations. Condoms are excellent for contraception and preventing sexually transmitted infections, but wearing a piece of latex over one's penis necessarily reduces the sensations experienced during intercourse. Many men complain they feel very little when wearing a condom, and this can interfere with achieving an orgasm. Among older couples, the man faces different challenges: he requires more stimulation to climax, while the woman's vagina, which has become more lax, provides less stimulation during sex. Many postmenopausal women require lubricants for sex, but too much can make the man feel like he's swimming in it. Some friction is a good thing!

None of these issues pertained to David. He was young and healthy, with a normal physical examination and normal levels of testosterone. The real clue to David's inability to climax during intercourse was when he said, "I just don't get the same kind of stimulation from sex that I do with masturbation."

I asked David what he remembered about the first time he ejaculated. He described being an eleven- or twelve-year-old boy on a hotel bed in Paris, on a family vacation. The bedsheets had a pleasant fragrance that struck him as very feminine, so different from the fragrances of home, and conjured up the enchanting scents he experienced as Parisian women walked by. He was lying facedown in his undershorts, with his body rubbing against the sheets. All of a sudden, he felt a strange warmth and discovered a sticky, creamy wet spot on the front of his shorts.

David still masturbated by rubbing himself against his sheets. Without realizing it, he had trained himself over the years to come with a kind of stimulation that was not replicated by a penis going in and out of a vagina, or even by oral sex. What brought him to orgasm was pressure against his scrotum and the underside of his penis. When David had sex, he usually insisted on being on top, face-to-face. He felt like he was more in control this way, and could show off his remarkable sexual endurance, pumping away as he'd seen in a porn video when he first became sexually active. David experienced pleasurable sensations this way; however, they didn't come close to bringing him to a climax. This was the crux of the problem. David needed a kind of stimulation to achieve orgasm that he wasn't getting from intercourse, or even oral sex.

I was confident David would be able to come during sex if he could discover a way to receive the kind of stimulation he needed. I made two suggestions. The first was to buy Sarah a fragrance that reminded him of Paris. Scents are powerful cues. Almost everyone can associate early memories with distinctive smells (e.g., Grandma's house). My idea was to bring David back to his primal sexual experience. David liked the idea when I explained it, but asked, "What if Sarah doesn't want to wear it?"

"Just have her try it on," I suggested, "put your arms around her, inhale deeply next to her ear, and tell her you feel like you're walking along the Seine, on a misty Sunday morning, with the most beautiful woman in the universe." He smiled broadly. It was a corny line, but he thought he could pull it off.

My second suggestion was to play a sexual game with Sarah, in which Sarah would be on top, with David's hands on her hips. Sarah was to move only under the guidance of David's hands. "Move her so that you feel pressure on the underside of your penis," I instructed. "And experiment with different speeds of moving back and forth. My guess is that you need a slower pace than what you've been doing. You're not a pumping machine!" If David could feel a physical sensation during intercourse that was similar to what he experienced on his own, I was certain he could find his way to an orgasm.

David seemed energized by the homework I'd given him. He was supposed to follow up with me in a few weeks but missed his appointment. Four months later my secretary informed me David had come to the office without an appointment, requesting to see me for a moment.

"Doctor, I have great news," he said. "Sarah and I are engaged!"

"David, that's wonderful. Congratulations!"

"Thank you. We've only told a few people so far, family and close friends, but I wanted you to know."

"I'm touched," I said truthfully. "Forgive me for asking, but I've been wondering about you. How did things go after our last visit together?"

"Everything worked out just like you predicted. I bought Sarah some expensive French perfume, she loved it and wore it the very same night, and when we made love I was so excited I came almost right away. We didn't even bother with that game you suggested. Sarah just picked up on what feels good for me, and I don't have any problem coming anymore."

Maybe Not So Rare After All

When I shared David's story with a friend in his early fifties, he told me that he had faked an orgasm himself on a few occasions.

"Really?" I asked incredulously.

"Sure. It's no big deal. Sometimes with my girlfriend I get the feeling that I'm not going to be able to come that night, especially if I've had any alcohol. After a while I pretend it happened, and then we both go to sleep."

I was stunned. After that, I began to ask some of my patients whether they ever faked an orgasm. The first few looked at me like I was nuts for asking such a ridiculous question. However, one man answered openly, "It's funny you ask. I've never told anyone this, but last year I became depressed after I sold my business, and my doctor prescribed an antidepressant. I'm off it now, but that medication made it really difficult for me to ejaculate. So a couple of times I faked it with my wife."

What Does Faking an Orgasm Tell Us About Men?

Apart from the surprise that a healthy young man might have difficulty achieving an orgasm with sex, and the curiosity as to how he pulled it off without Sarah suspecting, the real challenge posed by David is to our ideas about male sexual behavior.

If we take David's explanation at face value, he faked his orgasm for Sarah's benefit. Specifically, he wanted her to feel all right about herself as a sexually appealing, sexually capable woman. In that light, his gesture is considerate and kind. And in doing so, he risked losing Sarah. He was certain that Sarah would end the relationship if she discovered he'd been faking it. One could argue that David was simply acting in his own interest in order to keep his relationship going with Sarah. However, if trying to maintain a relationship is "selfish," who among us would be able to honestly plead "not guilty"?

Men want to be great partners. For a woman they care about they are willing to sacrifice themselves in any variety of ways. They may not always know the best course of action to take, and may act in ways that, from a woman's point of view, seem absurd or even counterproductive, but this does not diminish the motivation. That's why I like to say that a man's definition of *great sex* is when the woman says, "That was great sex."

3. THE FRETFUL PENIS, AND OTHER NATURAL REACTIONS TO UNFAIR EXPECTATIONS

There is no such thing as pure pleasure; some anxiety always goes with it.

—OVID (43 BC–AD 17), Roman poet

Barry's Performance Anxiety

"Doctor, I have trouble with my erections," Barry stated with considerable agitation. "One day my penis worked okay, and then suddenly it didn't." He wrung his hands together. Barry's hair was short, receding on the sides, and he combed it forward in the manner of a Roman emperor. He was forty-three years old, of average height and build, with very pale skin. He spoke English well despite a thick Russian accent. He worked in the town planning office of a local suburb and wore a white shirt and dress pants, with a purple tie that was a bit too wide and a bit too loud. He had been married for eleven years to Elsa, who was thirty-seven.

"Does your penis ever get hard anymore?" I asked.

"Yes!" he exclaimed with enthusiasm, as if he hoped this was a hopeful sign. "Yes, it does. Sometimes it is hard, sometimes soft. But even when it is hard, it doesn't last. What can I do?"

"Let's first see if we can figure out what's happening," I

answered. "You said that things changed suddenly. When did this happen?"

"About a month ago."

"And did anything special happen to you around that time? Did you start any new medicines, have any new treatments?"

"No. I don't take any medicines at all. Doctor, I'm a very healthy man. My father was seventy-eight when he died, and he still was having sex. This is why I don't understand what is happening to me."

"What about work? Are things all right there? Are you experiencing more stress lately? Less sleep?"

"Work is stressful. This is nothing new, though. It has always been this way."

"What about your relationship with Elsa?"

Barry didn't answer right away, as if he was debating whether to tell me something or not. Finally, he nodded his head and blurted out, "Elsa told me that I am too aggressive!"

I was quiet for a few moments to see if Barry wanted to say anything else. He was silent, though, just pursing his lips and tightening the muscles around his mouth and jaw, nodding his head as if he couldn't believe what had happened to him.

"When did Elsa say this to you?" I asked gently.

"About a month ago," he responded, but didn't seem to make the connection.

"And when she said you were too aggressive, what did she mean?"

"She said a lot of things. I'm not sure I understood it all. She said I act too suddenly and without thinking about her feelings. She told me she doesn't like it that I raise my voice to her. And she said her 'needs have changed' since we were first married."

"What did she mean by that?"

"She wants me to kiss her more. Talk to her more."

"Did she say you were too aggressive sexually?"

"I assume that was what she meant."

"You're not sure?"

Barry shrugged. "I assumed it."

"Okay, what has happened since you had that conversation?"

"Well, actually, the relationship is better," he said, his face and manner softening. "I'm trying. We talk more. Elsa is a good woman. Before, when I was stressed I would take it out on her because I thought she wouldn't understand my problems. Now, to tell the truth, when I tell her about work she sometimes makes a good suggestion. She looks happier. Everything is better except the sex."

"What happened there?"

"I didn't touch her for a while. Normally it is about twice a week. When we tried again, I couldn't get hard. I haven't had a good erection with Elsa since we had that conversation."

This was starting to make sense. The penis is not an automatic machine, capable of revving up at the slightest hint of sex. Oh sure, the early years of a boy's sexual awakening are characterized by too many erections, often at the most inopportune times (e.g., when riding on the school bus or being called up to the front of the class). And many of those early years are spent yearning for sex. Every opportunity to satisfy that hunger feels like a critical moment in our lives. Given how much men want sex, it seems almost incomprehensible that a man might experience a "power outage" when his partner is ready and willing.

It may be incomprehensible, but it's common. Young or old, men will find that their penis goes soft when their thoughts get ahead of them or when they're nervous. It's called performance anxiety. I wondered whether Barry was experiencing performance anxiety with Elsa.

We tend to think of erection and ejaculation as inextricably linked, with ejaculation the usual end point of the erection. Each has its own set of biological control mechanisms, though, including separate nerves. Ejaculation takes place when there has been sufficient arousal and stimulation. Normally, in a healthy man, that happens with a firm penis. However, the firmness of an erection depends on the action of blood vessels that respond to both

"Go!" and "Stop!" signals. The Go! signals are familiar enough, but anxiety and related negative thoughts stimulate the Stop! signals. Barry's ejaculation with a soft penis was one more clue that he was anxious, since anxiety often affects a man's erection more than his ability to ejaculate.

Barry told me that Elsa had never been very interested in sex but also hadn't complained about it. She was able to have an orgasm nearly every time, although this required direct stimulation of her clitoris, which the couple did together, her hand on top of his. Barry reported that his own erections with masturbation were normal, and he also woke in the morning on occasion with a firm erection that would stay firm until he urinated.

There are three and a half situations when grown men develop erections. One is with sex, of course. Another is with masturbation. And the third is upon awakening in the morning or night, often referred to by men as a *piss hard-on* because the penis is standing up when the man awakens to urinate. The "half" represents the spontaneous erection that occurs anytime, day or night, when a man has a sexual thought or sometimes for no good reason at all. I only give it half credit because these spontaneous erections tend to disappear in middle age.

As a rule, if the penis is able to get fully firm and stay firm during one of these occasions, it means that the mechanical aspects of erection work just fine. The only thing that can make an erection behave like a faulty wire is the mind.

A quick comment about men and masturbation: nearly all men do it, at least occasionally, but most feel guilty about it, as if the devil somehow got hold of their mind when they should have been doing something more productive. It's easy to imagine a man joining some buddies for beers on a weekend and bragging about the great sex he had recently. Can you imagine the same man sharing with gusto a story about masturbating to a great porn video clip? I don't think so. So it takes a certain, ahem, delicacy, to talk to men about masturbation.

Years ago, fresh out of my training and armed with the knowledge that a good sexual history was often the key to understanding a man and his problem, I marched straight ahead, blindly, into the world of masturbation. I asked men directly, "Do you masturbate?" as a preliminary question, wanting to follow up with whether or not the penis was hard when they were by themselves. I soon learned this was a *terrible* question. The most confident, articulate men would hem and haw, and become red in the face. Therefore, instead of asking men to "fess up to being a 'masturbator'" so that I could hear whether their solo erections were better than when they had sex with their partner, I came upon the idea of letting men assist me as problem solvers. Now, after hearing a story of lousy erections with sex, I ask, "Have you tried to see whether the same thing happens when you're by yourself?" To which men usually respond enthusiastically, "Sure, Doc! I had to take a look under the hood, if you know what I mean. Took it out for a test drive!" A world of men as wannabe auto mechanics.

Barry's normal erections with masturbation confirmed my suspicion that he was physically fine. His problem was psychological. In this case, and in most cases of psychological erectile dysfunction (ED), *psychological* doesn't necessarily mean that the person is odd or depressed or has deep-seated problems. It just means that the brain isn't working in concert with the body toward a sexually positive result. The most common psychological explanation for a story like Barry's is anxiety. Barry gave up the game when he added, "I'm panicked, Doctor. I don't know what to do."

Panic was a revealing word for Barry to use because it means anxiety taken to the extreme. I had no doubt that this was a true reflection of Barry's mental state when it came to having sex with Elsa.

Barry assumed that Elsa's comment that he was too rough with her referred to his sexual behavior, and he was left without a script to follow. Whatever he thought he was doing before now required reexamination. Uncertainty plus lack of confidence is an antiaphrodisiac. No wonder Barry was having trouble getting hard.

Barry surprised me with his next comment. "My wife said it would be okay if I had sex with other women, as long as she doesn't know about it." This didn't sound like something a woman would suggest.

"Barry, who suggested the idea of you sleeping with other women?" I asked.

"My wife."

"Why do you think she said that?"

"She knows sex is important to me and says it is not so important to her, so maybe I should find someone else to do it with. I haven't done it. I'm not interested. The person I want to be having sex with is my wife."

I love that part of the story. Barry, faced with a free pass from his wife to have sex outside the marriage without guilt, chose to not use it. The person he wants to have sex with is his own wife. How novel an idea!

Following Up with Barry

Barry came back to see me after we'd performed a number of tests. His original physical examination with me had been fine, and now his tests showed normal hormone levels, and the blood pressure and sensation in his penis were also normal. Perhaps most important, a useful test for rigidity, called a nocturnal penile tumescence (fullness) test (NPT for short), that measured Barry's sleeping erections showed that they were fine.

The NPT device consists of two bands which are placed on the penis when a man goes to bed at night, and he removes them in the morning. The bands are attached to a small monitor that measures every change in penile size and rigidity over the course of the night, and when the man returns the device to us, we download the information and obtain a graph showing what the penis "did" during the night.

Normal, healthy men usually have three to five erections each night, during the deepest part of sleep, lasting anywhere from five minutes to an hour or more. A single "event" with good rigidity that lasts ten minutes or more is as good a test as any that the penis has adequate blood flow and nerve function.

I showed Barry his NPT results, which revealed three erections the first night and four on the second night. The best erection was on the second night, with rigidity of 95 percent (anything above 70 percent is strongly suggestive of normal rigidity), lasting forty minutes.

"Barry, this is completely normal," I said. "When you're asleep and your mind isn't monitoring what's happening, your body is able to have firm, long-lasting erections. There's nothing wrong with your penis." Barry leaned back to process this information.

"Barry, it's time for you to talk to Elsa about sex," I continued. "You're afraid you're not doing it right for her, and the anxiety prevents your penis from becoming fully erect. Talk to her. You might be surprised to hear what she has to say."

"Doctor, I don't know how to talk to her about this. It's very embarrassing."

"Do you love Elsa?"

"What a question—of course!"

"Do you tell her you love her?"

"Sometimes."

"Okay. Start by telling her you love her, and that it matters very much to you to be able to have a sexual relationship that feels good for her. Be honest and tell her that you're afraid you haven't done a good job with her in the past."

"Doctor, I'll try."

Barry returned a couple of weeks later. "I spoke with Elsa," he said. "When I told her I didn't think I was good at sex with her, she told me she was afraid she wasn't good at sex for me! She was embarrassed she couldn't have an orgasm unless I touched her afterward. I never knew she felt that way! She said she really liked the way I touched her." Barry cleared his throat. "We had sex right away. Probably the best sex of my life. And now we're trying a couple of things, like touching Elsa before I go inside instead of after. It's actually fun doing it together now."

Country Sex

"Doctor, I can't get good erections," began Simon, a married small-business owner. "Sex has become a problem, and my wife is starting to complain."

"Tell me about it," I said.

"There's not much to tell you," he began. "I try to have sex with my wife, and my penis doesn't get hard. It's frustrating for me, and for her, obviously."

"Do you have a lot of stress?" I asked.

"Well, I've got a lot going on at work. The economy is killing me. I've done okay in the past, but I just can't keep carrying all my personnel if things don't improve soon, and some of my employees have been with me for years. It would kill me to let any of them go, but if I don't my business is going to run into the ground."

"You've got good reasons to be stressed," I said. "Let me ask you something. There must be times when you're less stressed than other times. I'm wondering if things are any different when you get away, perhaps on a vacation."

"Funny you mention that. I haven't taken a real vacation in years, but my wife and I do go up to our country house every weekend. You know what? Sex is fine when we're there."

"I'm wondering what is different for you between the country and the city."

"Doctor, they're totally different. During the week in the city, I'm always fielding phone calls, always stressed, I don't sleep well. And the country house"—his face lit up—"the country house is my refuge. I feel less and less stressed just making the two-hour drive on the highway." A thought seemed to dawn on Simon, and he asked, "You don't think this is stress-related, do you, Doctor?"

"It's certainly possible. What do you think?" I replied.

Simon almost started laughing. "Doctor, that's almost too obvious! Can stress really interfere with erections like that?"

"Stress can definitely interfere with erections. Stress, anxiety, depression, pain—all sorts of things can get in the way for a man."

"Well, why didn't I ever have those problems when I was younger, then?"

"My guess is that when you were twenty or twenty-five, you weren't the boss and worrying about letting go of valued employees."

"That's true."

"And as we age we lose some of our 'reserve power.' When we're young, our erections are more efficient, and even if there is something bothering us a bit, the excitement and anticipation of sex usually can overcome it. Once we're older, though, the balance between 'Yes, sex!' and 'No, I'm stressed!' shifts.

"Men often say that their penis has 'betrayed' them when they find they can't have sex. Actually, your penis is just reflecting what's going on in your mind and body. When it won't get hard, it is as if your penis is telling you, 'Something is wrong. I'm not feeling sexual.'"

"That makes sense," said Simon.

On his way into the exam room before I'd met him, Simon had asked my medical assistant if there was a possibility he might leave the same day with a prescription for one of the ED pills. During our visit, I had offered Simon a sample of one of the pills, but he wasn't interested.

"Thanks, but I'm good, Doc," he replied. "I think I just wanted to understand what was going on with me." Simon left the office happy. When he was stressed and preoccupied, he was unable to have sex. When he was more relaxed and his mind was freed from obsessing over the details of his work life, he was just fine. The connection between the two may seem obvious, but this was new information for Simon.

Not as Young as He Used to Be

"Doctor, something is terribly wrong," said Reuben, forty-eight. "My penis doesn't get hard enough, and it won't stay hard. I'm certain there's a blockage down there, in the penis or prostate."

"Tell me what happens when you have sex," I asked.

"I'm divorced," he told me, "and I'm dating a woman right now. Her name is Helen. She is about my age, she's in great shape, and she's *very* sexy. I do what I can for her, but nothing is working properly."

I try to be very specific with my questions about sex, breaking things down into their component parts. "What exactly is it that's not right?"

"I told you. My penis doesn't get hard like it used to, it won't stay hard, and there's a blockage down there."

"Okay, I hear you. Your erection doesn't get hard like it used to, it doesn't stay hard like it used to, and you believe there is a blockage. Reuben, I'd like to try to get more specific, so please humor me. Is that okay?"

He nodded yes.

"How often do you and Helen get together?"

"About three times a week."

One of the most functional, practical distinctions for men with erection problems is whether or not their penis achieves sufficient rigidity to penetrate the vagina. It takes a fair amount of rigidity to do so. "Are you ever able to put your penis inside Helen's vagina when you have sex?"

"Sure. But it's not like before."

"Okay, it's not like before. What I'm trying to understand is this: if you and Helen got together ten different times, how many of those ten times would you be able to go inside?"

"Every time," he answered, as if I were missing his point. "What I'm telling you is it's not the same." I nodded to indicate I understood it wasn't the same. At least we were getting somewhere.

"And when you say the penis won't stay hard, does it soften before you have an orgasm?" I asked.

"No, I stay hard until I come."

This was confusing. "So when does it soften?"

"A lot of the time."

"Can you explain when it happens?"

"When we're having sex!" he said, exasperated with me.

Obviously, I wasn't getting something. I decided to change topics.

"Why don't you tell me about the blockage," I suggested.

Reuben was clearly quite disturbed about some changes he'd noticed. I wasn't sure why he believed he had a blockage, but it was certainly true that blockages of the arteries leading to the penis can cause ED.

"Why do you think you have a blockage?" I asked.

"It's obvious," Reuben insisted. "When I was married, the fluid would squirt out whenever I came. Not anymore. Now it oozes out. In fact, some of it can ooze out a long time after I'm done. Five to ten minutes later. If that's not a blockage, then I don't know what is."

I was starting to understand. "Reuben, how long ago did your marriage end?"

"Six years ago."

"Have you had sex since then with any partners other than Helen?"

"No, Helen is the first."

"And how long have you two been dating?"

"About three months." This was making even more sense now.

"Reuben, when you and Helen get together, do you try to have sex more than once?"

"Of course."

"So are you telling me that the first time you do it, everything is fine, the penis gets hard and stays hard until you're finished, but the penis won't get fully hard or stay completely hard the second time around?"

"That's what I've been trying to tell you," he said, more with exasperation than satisfaction at my delayed comprehension.

I had an idea. "Excuse me, Reuben. I'll be right back."

A few minutes later I returned to Reuben's exam room with the Pillars of Hardness, as I like to call it. The Pillars is a simple yet brilliant tool. It consists of four rubber cylinders, each about four to five inches in length and an inch in diameter, pointing straight up. Moving from left to right, each of these four cylinders has increasing firmness, corresponding to values 1 through 4. The one on the far left, labeled #1, is spongy, fully compressible, and can be bent in half without any effort at all, like a penis that has fullness but no firmness. In contrast, #4 on the far right is hard; it has almost no give when squeezed along the sides of the cylinder, and it cannot be bent. Hardnesses #3 and #4 are considered normal erections, more than adequate for intercourse, whereas it would be difficult to have sex with a penis that has the hardness of #1.

If a man tells me that his erection isn't as hard as it used to be, it can be difficult to know how much of a problem we're dealing with. The beauty of the Pillars is that patient and physician can have a common source of comparison to assess rigidity. I showed the Pillars to Reuben and asked him to feel each one in turn.

"Which one is most like the firmness you have the first time you have sex with Helen?" I asked.

"This one," he replied, pointing to #4—fully hard.

"And which one is most like your penis when you say it has lost its rigidity?"

"This one." He pointed to #3—almost fully hard. This was making sense now. The second time Reuben and Helen had sex on a given evening, Reuben's erection was still pretty firm, just not as firm as the first one.

There were a couple of loose ends I needed to tie up. "Reuben, does Helen complain that your penis is too soft?" I asked.

"Not at all. If she's bothered by it, she hasn't said anything. Actually, she seems to be quite happy with the sex we're having."

I performed an examination, which was entirely normal, and we sat down together to talk things through. "Reuben, what would you like to come from this visit?"

"I want you to figure out what is causing this blockage and fix it for me."

"I'm pleased to tell you that I don't think there is anything worrisome happening with you." Reuben did not seem nearly as pleased. "What you've been describing are the things that happen normally to men as they get older. It's quite normal for the second erection to be less firm than the first. In fact, you're quite fortunate to be able to go two rounds at age forty-eight. I have plenty of patients your age who struggle to have sex even once." Reuben was unmoved. "The good news for you is that you're almost fifty, you still have a very functional penis, and a very active sex life. You should be happy!" I said, trying to reframe his complaints in a more positive light.

"Doctor, that seems highly unlikely. What about my blockage?"

"Reuben, it's normal as we age for the semen to come out with less force. It still comes out, but more slowly, and the last few drops usually just ooze out over time. It's not a sign of a blockage."

Reuben and I spoke a little longer, but he wasn't having any of it, and his expression as he left the office indicated he thought he'd wasted his time. He was convinced that the changes he'd noticed indicated a problem, and no amount of explaining on my part was going to change his mind.

His sexual functioning was still very good, just not as good as he'd expected. Helen didn't seem to have a problem with it. It had been confusing to me when Reuben referred to his erections being less hard when he was so easily able to have sex "every time," but this was a relative thing. The tipoff for me was the description of the changes in ejaculation. Many men bring this up. It may seem like a blockage if a man expects the semen to shoot out like a fifteen-year-old, hitting the ceiling light if precautions weren't taken, but the loss of power with ejaculation is merely a reflection of a more lax urethra (the passageway within the penis and prostate for urine and semen) and some enlargement of the prostate. Men will often notice that if it has been a longer time than usual since their last sexual episode, or if they are especially aroused, the fluid will come out with more force.

The irony of Reuben's story is that he worked as an actuary for an insurance company, assessing the impact of age on the risk of death and disability. It was his *business* to recognize how much age affects our health, yet he was blind to the effects of age on sexual function. It's not Reuben's fault. Where does this information exist? In the movies we often see increasingly older leading men get the girl, with no sense that their sexual powers may not be quite what they were when they were twenty-one. Given what I've seen over the years, though, my own reflex as I sit in the theater is to say to myself, "I hope he brought along some Viagra!"

Like women, men can be fussy about the conditions under which they like sex, whether physical or psychological. But for a man, an obstacle in either realm can be devastating. Some of this has to do with unrealistic expectations about our physical abilities, particularly as we age. Just like the forty-five-year-old, 280-pound couch potato who gets winded from walking up a single flight of stairs but who insists he is still an athlete because he played on a varsity team in high school, men seem to believe their sexual powers also do not diminish. If only it were true. Most fifteen-year-old boys are able to achieve a full, firm erection on the worst day of their lives. Many fifty-five-year-old, perfectly healthy men will be unable to get an erection at all if they have one important, uncompleted item on their to-do list.

In their teen years and early twenties, young men may be unaware that an erection can be partially firm. At that age, either the erection is there or it isn't—up or down, yes or no. This response changes as men move into their thirties and beyond. Simon's case was a good example of how our lack of knowledge regarding real male sexuality is a bigger problem than we think it is.

Barry's story is a great example of how important a conversation can be. We all have our own ideas about sex and our own sexuality, but the topic is so private, feels so personal, that it's difficult to discuss even with a long-term partner. Am I doing okay? Does he/she find me sexy? We look for clues, hints, and try to not be too obvious that we care so much.

With ads everywhere for Viagra and Cialis and graphic descriptions of sexual positions in *Cosmo* and *Playboy*, we are in an age of ubiquitous information about sex. There has never been a time in history like this. Yet the private, personal, emotional part of sex is still too intimate for many couples to talk about. Most of us, men and women, still experience some degree of shame, guilt, and uncertainty about our sexuality. And with the absence of realistic information about male sexuality in particular, we are left with ample room for misunderstandings that can impact our ability to have loving, satisfying relationships.

We all have ideas about what sex is and what it should be. How it should look, what it should feel like. But sometimes those ideas are all based on fantasies and romantic notions. The analytical among us try to distill information from our human experiences and combine that with what we read and see in the media as the "right way" for sex to be. The problem is that so much of this is wrong.

I believe that sex is an important part of relationships and one of the keys to real intimacy in a relationship. For a lot of men, it is the *only* way they experience and contribute to intimacy. Moreover, women are not alone in having overly romantic or unrealistic ideas about what sex should be like. Here's the big picture as I see it. A man's ability to have sex is a complicated and delicate process, and any number of problems may cause a man's equipment to fail, including stress and anxiety. It is important to recognize that as a man ages, his physical responsiveness and abilities change too, and moreover, he becomes increasingly vulnerable to physical causes of ED. That's reality. Sex at fifty or sixty or seventy may not be what it was at twenty-five, and at that age a man may require a pill or some other assistance, but sex still remains a critical part of how we find fulfillment in relationships.

Recently, Homer, eighty-three and a widower, came to see me for an annual visit. His medications included Cialis and testosterone. I asked if he was having sex these days.

"Oh yes," he replied. "I feel very fortunate. I've been dating a lovely woman in her seventies. And believe it or not, I'm having the best sex of my life!"

May we all feel that way at eighty-three.

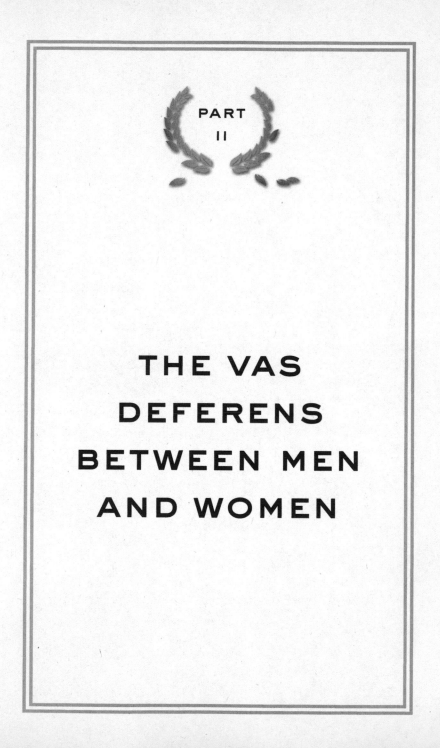

PART
II

THE VAS
DEFERENS
BETWEEN MEN
AND WOMEN

4. WHAT IS A MAN?

*I've always felt that sexuality is a really slippery thing.
In this day and age, it tends to get categorized and
labeled, and I think labels are for food. Canned food.*

—MICHAEL STIPE, lead singer, R.E.M.

There are some things in life that don't seem to require explanation. One of these is gender. Little children don't need to ask
whether Uncle Harry is a boy or a girl, and it is usually immediately obvious when they meet other children whether they are dealing with a boy or girl like themselves or a child of the opposite sex.

The distinction between the sexes is quite obvious, isn't it?
Even the term *opposite sex* carries with it the implication that
males and females are polar extremes. In our own culture and in
many others, we make important distinctions between men and
women, with regard to laws, employment, societal roles, athlet-
ics, religion, and also within relationships. We may all be human,
yet we act as if males and females were two different species
populating the same biosphere that have somehow become inter-
dependent.

From our youngest years we learn that men and women are not
only anatomically different from each other but also biologically

and psychologically distinct. Books like *Men Are from Mars, Women Are from Venus* confirm what we already believe about the oh-so-different ways that men and women behave and think, and engage in relationships.

To me, it's not quite so simple. There *are* important distinctions between men and women, but I believe we've gone much too far in asserting those differences. From a biological perspective, perhaps even a medical perspective, and well, gosh-darn it, from a Dr. Abe perspective, what is striking is not so much the *differences* between the sexes but the *similarities*. If you and I are to share these pages as reader and writer, contemplating the world of male sexuality, then it is necessary for me to lay things out as I see them. And the key question to get us started is this: what is a man?

French Toast Pistol

Some years ago as I waited to pick up my daughter from preschool, I chatted with Claudia, the mother of a boy in the same class, about the differences between boys and girls. We had been watching with amusement as the boys ran around the play space, in some cases literally bouncing off the walls and each other, while a group of girls sat together with their tiny doll-sized cups and saucers enjoying an imaginary tea party.

"I've always believed that culture has an enormous impact on human behavior," Claudia said, "and was convinced that aggression in boys was learned, and came from things like television shows and bad family experiences. So when my son Jacob was born, my husband and I got rid of our TV set and were careful that no books or toys associated with any kind of violence would come into the house, not even a water pistol." She sighed. "Then one day, out of the blue, Jacob grabbed a piece of French toast off his plate, folded it into a gun, and started 'shooting' at our dog and anything else that moved." Claudia laughed. "All my beliefs, out the window! There's no question about it—the differences between boys and girls must be biological. Must be all that darn testosterone!"

One needn't be a professor of anthropology to recognize that boys and girls behave differently. Yet Claudia was surprised when I informed her that little boys and girls have the same amount of testosterone. For both of them, testosterone levels are so low as to be almost undetectable. Claudia was also right, though, that testosterone does explain some of the behavioral differences between boys and girls. Early in a boy's life, there are two transient bursts of testosterone that tell the genitalia to develop in a male form—penis instead of clitoris, scrotum instead of labia—and that also are believed to imprint a male pattern on the brain. From shortly after birth until puberty, however, the testicles are quiet, making no more testosterone than a female child would have. And then at puberty, watch out! The testicles begin to produce the large amounts of testosterone that will mark an individual as a male forever.

Misinformation of the sort Claudia displayed is near-universal. This superficial level of knowledge is like the tourist who says he "knows" New York City because he has visited Times Square. Not only does Times Square fail to capture the remarkable variety and essence of New York, but even more, the impression that Times Square *does* represent New York creates a more misleading picture than if one had never been to Times Square at all.

So it is with men. The two-dimensional portrayal of men in the popular media, thriving exclusively on sex, food, sports, and violence, has created countless layers of false "knowledge" about what men are like. The thousands of men who have passed through my examination room over more than twenty years of practice have dropped not only their trousers for me but also their public masks.

"I Came to America to Become a Man"

Early in my career a young man was brought to my clinic by four of his brothers. Effie had arrived in the States a few weeks earlier from a western African nation, and spoke no English, so his eldest brother translated. Effie was twenty-one and had been born without testicles. His brother explained that Effie had been happy in his life back home and reluctant to join his brothers in Boston, despite their exhortations to emigrate. The winning argument came when the oldest brother told Effie that U.S. surgeons could probably give him testicles. Effie wanted "balls," the brother explained. When friends and family asked Effie why he had finally agreed to come to the United States, he answered, "I came to America to become a man."

With his brother translating, Effie told his story. He had a pleasant, almost handsome rectangular face, framed by short, tightly curled hair, and a carefully trimmed beard. He had a winning, toothy smile, and his eyebrows rose and fell as he talked. I had the impression he could be very funny, if only I understood his language.

When Effie was born, his parents discovered he was missing his testicles. The doctors told them the testicles were inside his body and might come down on their own with enough time. When he was five years old and the testicles hadn't descended, the doctors told Effie's parents to return when he was older. When he was nine and still had no visible testicles, the doctors' advice was to return when he was a teenager. At fifteen he was told he was too old for the doctors to do anything.

Despite his apparent lack of testicles, Effie went through an otherwise normal puberty and early adulthood. He had worked as a laborer. Over the years he had several girlfriends with whom he'd experienced successful sexual intercourse, complete with ejaculation. He had no complaints about his health, other than feeling incomplete as a man without testicles.

On examination, there was no reason to doubt that Effie was a man. His body was lean and muscular. He had no breast tissue, and his penis was entirely normal in size and girth. However, the scrotum was empty. The scrotum itself, the sac that normally contains the testicles, was unusually small and lay tight against his body, as if to confirm that it had never contained anything. I examined the inguinal region, the area just above the crease between leg and abdomen, where most undescended testicles are found, but I felt nothing.

Based on his appearance, I was certain that Effie had at least one testicle somewhere. The testicles are responsible for 95 percent of testosterone production (the adrenals produce the remaining 5 percent), and the only way an individual can become completely virilized like Effie is with substantial concentrations of testosterone. With no testicles palpable within the inguinal regions, the most likely location of Effie's testicle or testicles was deep within his abdomen.

The Incredible Journey

Early in fetal life the testicles sit inside the body, adjacent to the kidneys, and gradually descend, finally emerging into the inguinal canal on their way to the scrotum somewhere around the eighth fetal month. It is an incredible journey. Indeed, the testicles win the prize for the greatest distance traveled during normal development. Embryologists have been debating for decades how the testicles make their descent into the scrotum. One theory holds that the testicles are pulled down by a fibrous attachment connecting the lower pole of the testicles to the scrotum, called the gubernaculum. Another argues that the migration of the testicles is not really a migration at all. Rather, the testicles stay right where they are, but every other structure around them grows asymmetrically in an upward direction, making it seem that the testicles are descending.

During descent, the testicles invert a layer of the peritoneum, the membrane holding our abdominal contents in place, to form an extra coat around itself and then must locate the special point in the lower abdominal wall, called the inguinal canal, where they emerge from the abdomen on their way to the scrotum. How does the abdominal wall know to allow the testicles to pass through? In my perhaps overly fervent imagination, I envision the testicles tapping along the inside part of the abdominal wall, listening for the hollow sound that will indicate the secret panel that will open the door to a hidden passageway. Once through the muscle, however, this passageway remains forever a point of potential weakness in the abdominal wall and is the spot where most hernias occur later in life.

Given the length and complexity of this journey, it should not be surprising that some testicles don't make it all the way into the scrotum. Approximately 1 percent of boys are born with one or both testicles undescended, a condition called cryptorchidism. Some testicles do manage to drop down spontaneously within the first year of life, but these are usually the ones that had only a short distance to go, lying near the upper part of the scrotum at birth.

There are a few worrisome aspects of undescended testicles. For one, they are at increased risk of developing cancer. And since the undescended testicle cannot be palpated, it is impossible to feel for an early tumor. A second problem is that testicles exposed too long to the warmer temperature of the inguinal canal or abdomen lose their ability to produce sperm. By two years there are already irreversible changes in the undescended testicle that make it less likely for the individual to be fertile later in life. Finally, there is the cosmetic issue. Imagine what kids might say to another boy who is discovered to only have one testicle. Or none at all.

For these reasons, in the United States there is generally an urgency to operate on boys with undescended testicles early in life. When I was in my training, rotating through the renowned Children's Hospital of Boston, surgery for cryptorchidism was delayed until the boys were at least two years old and could more easily withstand the effects of anesthesia. Today, with improved pediatric anesthesia, surgery is performed at one year, or even earlier in some cases.

One Testicle or Two?

Before agreeing to operate on Effie, I needed to make sure I knew more about what I was dealing with. A CT scan identified two testicles lying within the lower part of the abdomen. Blood tests indicated normal levels of male hormones, including testosterone. A semen analysis showed a normal amount of fluid but no sperm. For completeness I obtained a karyotype, which revealed the normal chromosome pattern for a male, 46XY.

Effie wanted me to bring his testicles into his scrotum for one reason only: he wanted to feel like a man. However, there were a number of medical issues to consider. First, there was no guarantee that I'd be able to bring down even one of his testicles. The main determinant would be whether the blood vessels feeding and draining the testicles would be long enough to allow the testicles to reach all the way into the scrotum. If I tried to make the testicles reach too far, their blood supply could be compromised, and the testicles would atrophy. Effie's abdominal testicles were making adequate amounts of testosterone; if the testicles didn't survive, he would need testosterone treatment for the rest of his life.

Another issue was the increased risk of cancer. Removing both testicles would be safest from a cancer perspective, but this obviously was not what Effie was looking for. At least he could perform self-examinations of his testicles if they were brought down, and let his doctor know if he felt a lump. Finally, there was the fertility issue. It was important to let Effie know that he was making no sperm, and that even if I were to bring down both testicles successfully, there was no serious hope of producing sperm, or offspring, in the future.

I met with Effie and his brothers one last time before setting the date for surgery to discuss these various issues. I also mentioned that I could place a testicular implant, a fake testicle, on one or both sides if I couldn't bring down his own. This precipitated a conversation between Effie and several of his brothers.

The eldest turned to me. "Doctor, Effie says he doesn't want anything artificial. Besides, he likes you. He is certain you will be successful." Effie was grinning at me.

"What's This?"

At surgery, once Effie was anesthetized I opened his abdomen through a vertical incision from his pubic bone to his navel, and immediately found two fine-looking testicles, floating happily inside him. Yet something about the appearance of the pelvis struck me as female, with the two testicles in the usual location for ovaries. In fact, in that location, the testicles *looked* like ovaries. While I evaluated them for possible malignancy, my resident for the case looked deeper into the pelvis.

"Dr. Morgentaler!" he exclaimed, "What's this?" he asked, as he pulled up something unusual from the depths of the pelvis with a clamp. It was triangular, with the broad part toward the head, tapering down toward the feet. It didn't seem possible, but there it was. A uterus! It was small yet fully formed, just as one would find in a girl prior to puberty.

Investigating further, we discovered the testicles were attached to the uterus via a broad ligament, typical of the normal attachments of the ovaries to the uterus. And running along the top of the broad ligament were Fallopian tubes, the structure through which a female's eggs travel from the ovary to the uterus, and the place where sperm usually meet the egg and fertilize it.

Effie had two testicles, two vasa deferentia (the tubes that carry sperm from the testicles), one uterus, and two Fallopian tubes. Incredible! Except for the absence of ovaries, Effie had a complete set of male *and* female reproductive structures. It was now clear why the testicles had failed to descend properly; they were attached to the uterus and Fallopian tubes.

Now that I knew what we were dealing with, it was time to go to work. I transected the uterus at its base and removed it together with the Fallopian tubes. I then freed up both testicles from their attachments, taking care to preserve the delicate blood vessels. There was pretty good length of the blood vessels on both sides, with slightly greater length on the right side. With the testicles freed up like this, they looked like yo-yos at the end of a thick string.

Next I created a small gap in the abdominal wall on each side, as low toward the pubic bone as possible, through which I gently prodded and pulled on the testicles. The trick was to create an opening large enough to allow the testicles to pass through, but not so large as to allow fat or intestine to work their way through later, creating a hernia.

Both testicles came through well, and the blood vessels still seemed to be long enough for the testicles to reach the scrotum. So far so good. Next, with my fingers I pushed apart tissues in the inguinal region and into the scrotum, creating a pathway for the testicles to follow. The poor scrotum, empty for twenty-one years, did not immediately appear receptive to the idea of gaining new tenants. Slowly, and with care to not tear the skin, I stretched the scrotum to a size that would readily accept a testicle on each side.

The testicles were free and mobile. I placed them on top of the scrotum to make sure they would reach. The right one was fine, but the left one only reached to the top of the scrotum; nothing I did gave it enough length. I placed the right testicle into the scrotum, and it sat happily at the bottom of the sac, artery clearly pulsing, color good. I tried placing the left testicle into the scrotum. When I gently pulled it down where it belonged, it turned dusky. Released, a healthier color returned, but it rose to an awkward location where the leg joined the body. The left testicle was in a no-man's-land (a very appropriate term!); it wouldn't survive in the scrotum, and it would be a constant source of discomfort if I left it higher up. Moreover, if I couldn't get it down into the scrotum where it could be examined easily, Effie would require a lifetime of X-rays to make sure this testicle didn't develop cancer. I removed the left testicle.

Two Sets of Equipment

What had happened to Effie biologically that would result in his having a uterus?

We are born into this world as boys or girls, yet we don't start out this way. Until the eighth week of fetal life the anatomy of boys and girls is identical. We begin with an undifferentiated gonad that will eventually become either a testicle or an ovary. Until that time, all of us have both sets of rudimentary structures that are destined to mature into the reproductive system for one sex or the other. One set is called the Wolffian ducts, and under the influence of testosterone these will become the male structures of epididymis, vas deferens, and seminal vesicles. The other is called the Müllerian ducts, and these develop into vagina, uterus, and Fallopian tubes. We begin to have an inkling of what happened to Effie once we recognize that every fetus begins with both Wolffian and Müllerian ducts.

In boys, genes on the Y chromosome turn the gonad into a testicle, which then secretes two critical substances at key moments. One is testosterone, which influences the Wolffian ducts to mature into the male structures mentioned above. The other is called anti-Müllerian factor, and its job, as its name suggests, is to cause the Müllerian structures to regress. Two small remnants of the Müllerian ducts persist in adult men. One is a tiny appendage next to the testicle, of no consequence. The other sits within the prostatic portion of the urethra (the urine passageway), appearing as a small mound. Its name? The utricle. Tiny uterus.

So what happened to Effie? His Müllerian duct structures never regressed. Indeed, his pathology report later described a completely normal juvenile uterus. Effie's official diagnosis was Persistent Müllerian Duct Syndrome. It is very rare, as one can imagine. The curious aspect of these cases is why the Müllerian structures don't disappear as they should. After surgery, I sent Effie's blood to a research laboratory studying anti-Müllerian factor. Effie had normal adult levels, which was puzzling. Perhaps his body had begun secreting anti-Müllerian factor too late during development, or it was a mutated nonfunctional form, or his tissues failed to recognize the signal properly. We will never know the complete explanation.

Some readers will wonder what the presence of a uterus and Fallopian tubes says about Effie as a man. Effie had a normal male karyotype, with a Y chromosome. He had a penis and testicles, even if the latter were in an abnormal location. He had normal male levels of testosterone. He looked like a man, felt like a man, and behaved like a man. He just happened to have a uterus that had refused to leave the stage when given its cue. Men and women are physically much more similar than they appear. Both start with the same basic equipment. It is only the influence of hormones and other chemical signals that differentiate them.

"Man Gets Himself Pregnant!"

One of the most common questions my students ask when I present Effie's case is whether he was a hermaphrodite. Another question is whether he could have impregnated himself, since he had both testicles and a uterus.

In Greek mythology, Hermaphroditos was the son of the gods Hermes and Aphrodite, rendered in Greco-Roman art as possessing both breasts and male genitals. During a trip to the Louvre in Paris a few years ago, I stumbled upon a beautiful statue of Hermaphroditos. From the main passageway a few paces away, one sees a lovely woman reclining, the left leg rising upward bent at the knee, breasts partly exposed under a diaphanous gown. Only upon moving to the other side of the statue does one see a penis emerging from under the gown, initially hidden by the partially upraised leg.

Tabloids love the idea of a hermaphrodite, a he-she that in theory could self-impregnate, even though there are no documented cases where this has actually happened. Yet the idea of some mixture of male and female has captured our imagination for millennia.

We are fascinated by things that challenge our basic ideas of the world, and what could be more challenging than an individual with both male and female parts?

Technically, Effie was not a true hermaphrodite, which is defined by the presence of both gonads—that is, testicles and ovaries. Those cases are exceedingly rare. Since Effie only had one type of gonad, namely testicles, he is considered a pseudohermaphrodite. As for impregnating oneself, the hormonal conditions that allow sperm to be produced are anathema to the conditions that would allow eggs development and fertilization to take place. By the same token, the high estrogen concentrations necessary for egg development by the ovary would suppress sperm production.

How to Tell a Man He Was Born with a Uterus

On the day after surgery I walked into Effie's hospital room, where, as always, he was surrounded by his brothers. When I spoke to Effie, the eldest brother translated, and everyone paid attention. I told Effie that I had found the reason his testicles had not descended properly at birth. I said that within Effie's pelvis were structures that should have disappeared before birth, but remained, and had interfered with the ability of the testicles to drop into the scrotum. I explained that I had removed them. I never used the word *uterus*. There was a general nodding of understanding and appreciation of this information by Effie and his brothers, and I left the room with all of them celebrating my report that the one testicle appeared healthy in the scrotum.

At Effie's follow-up visit a month later, his right testicle was healthy, and his hormone levels were good. He was delighted. And he had a gift for me. In two medium-sized boxes filled with shredded newspaper were a pair of giant ostrich eggs, each with a little display stand. A small hole at the poles of each egg had been used to drain the contents. Effie's brother explained that in their country this was a traditional gift of honor and gratitude. I was touched. However, my immediate reaction upon seeing the two eggs unwrapped was how much these looked like two giant testicles! How fitting to receive such a gift from someone born with an empty scrotum who had traveled halfway around the world to satisfy his wish to feel like a man.

The Woman Who Wanted a Vasectomy Reversal

Darla was forty-six, tall, with soft, blond, wavy shoulder-length hair. Her bright blue eyeshadow was slightly smudged above her left eye, and I suspected she was wearing false eyelashes, although I couldn't be sure. Her husband, Eric, thirty-seven, was slender, with a full beard. He was handsome, with delicate facial features, like a darker version of a young Brad Pitt.

"I'd like to have my vasectomy reversed," Darla told me.

It took me a moment to process this request. "Okay," I said. "Why don't you tell me your story."

"Well, it's pretty simple, really. Eric and I would like to have a child, but I had a vasectomy when I was younger. We were told you were an expert at vasectomy reversal, so here we are."

"I take it that you were born as a man," I ventured.

"Actually," Darla answered, "it took me about seventeen years to become a *man*"—she exchanged a smile with Eric—"but I *was* born male, if that's what you mean."

"Right." I smiled. "So how did you decide to have a vasectomy?"

"I was married at the time. And my wife and I had a son. When he was about six years old, I realized I didn't want to have any more children. So I had a vasectomy."

"So you were living at the time as a man?" I asked.

"Oh yes," replied Darla.

"And how long have you been living as a woman?"

"It's been over ten years now."

I now noticed that Darla had traces of beard stubble over a somewhat prominent jawline. She was wearing a white silk blouse, unbuttoned far enough to reveal just the very tops of what appeared to be medium-sized breasts. A patterned skirt fell to just below her knees, and tan high heels completed her outfit.

"Have you had any surgery for your transition to being a woman?"

"No surgery," Darla replied, "other than the vasectomy. My only treatment has been with hormones. I take a medicine called spironolactone to block the effects of testosterone, and I take estrogen. The estrogen helped my breasts develop."

"They're really quite nice," added Eric, speaking for the first time. "Darla's breasts, I mean," he added.

I was beginning to understand Darla's situation a bit more clearly. "How long ago did you have the vasectomy performed?" I asked. The time that has elapsed since a vasectomy can influence the success of the reversal.

"It's been twelve years now," said Darla.

"And if the vasectomy reversal is successful, do you have someone lined up who would use the sperm to become pregnant?"

"Of course!"

"Were you planning to use a surrogate?"

"A surrogate?" Darla voice rose in indignation. Eric seemed disturbed by my question too. "Why would we need a surrogate? The whole point of the vasectomy reversal is to get Eric pregnant!"

Wow!

"Eric," I asked, "I gather, then, that you were born female?"

"That's right, Doctor," he answered.

"You want to get pregnant with sperm from Darla?"

"Right."

"And have you undergone any surgery?"

"Yes. I had my breasts removed, but no work done down below. My doctor tells me that everything down there should be able to function normally. I'm turning thirty-eight in a few months, though, so my biological clock is ticking. That's why Darla and I want to get going with this now. Once Darla has her reversal, how long do you think it will take for me to get pregnant?"

This was complicated. Darla was born a man, lived as a woman, and wanted her vasectomy reversed. Eric was born a woman but lived as a man, and wanted to become pregnant. Technically, there was no reason I couldn't perform a vasectomy reversal on Darla, with a strong likelihood of success. However, a major problem was that both Darla and Eric were taking hormones that prevented their reproductive organs from functioning properly. If Darla wanted to make sperm, she would need to stop her hormones for a minimum of six months. Eric would also need to stop taking his hormones to become pregnant, and for the duration of the pregnancy. I wondered whether Darla and Eric were prepared for this.

I asked Darla to lie down on the exam table. I paused for a moment, considering whether I needed to bring in a female assistant as a chaperone, a routine procedure when a male physician examines a woman, but decided it wasn't necessary in this case. Darla unzipped her skirt and slid it down to her knees. And there was revealed a perfectly normal but totally out-of-place set of male genitalia. Darla had a completely normal penis, a scrotum, and two testicles. The testicles were smaller than usual, from the hormonal treatments, but were otherwise fine. On the right and left sides I was able to feel the vas deferens, the tube that was cut during the vasectomy. There was a small gap between the two ends on each side from the procedure.

As I was finishing up my exam, I asked Darla, "Have you ever had your prostate checked?"

"Oh sure," said Darla. "My gynecologist checks it regularly." This was too funny! I couldn't help but wonder if I was being secretly videotaped for a reality television show.

"The technical part of the vasectomy reversal is fairly straightforward," I explained when Darla had dressed. "The likelihood of a successful procedure in your case—meaning that the tubes are put together so that sperm can come out with ejaculation—is about eighty percent in my hands."

Darla and Eric exchanged happy glances.

"We didn't expect the chances to be so good," said Eric.

"Well, let me be clear. A successful vasectomy reversal doesn't mean a pregnancy," I explained. "Even when a man has great sperm numbers, that's not always enough to guarantee a pregnancy. The woman may have her own issues with getting pregnant."

"That's okay," Darla said excitedly. "If you can get sperm to come out of me, then we should be all set, because Eric's doctor says he shouldn't really have any trouble getting pregnant."

"It's not so simple," I said.

"Why not?" Darla asked.

"There are a few issues. Darla, you're not making any sperm right now because of the hormone treatments. I could do a perfect operation, the tubes could be wide open, but there are no sperm to come out. If I did the reversal, you would need to go off the hormones for six months, maybe longer, while you're trying to make a baby. Are you willing to do that?"

"I guess so," replied Darla, "if that's what it will take." She didn't seem happy.

"And you, Eric, will also need to go off hormones while you're trying to become pregnant. And you can't be on male hormones once you are pregnant."

"My doctor didn't tell me that!" Eric replied, a bit of panic in his voice. "Darla, I can't come off my hormones," he said.

"Eric, let me ask you something. What will it be like for you, as a man, to get pregnant? How will you handle that at work?"

"I've thought this through," Eric said, gathering himself. "I work in an office. Customer support at a software company out on Route 128," he said, referring to the highway ringing Boston that housed hundreds of high-tech businesses, Boston's equivalent of Silicon Valley. "No one suspects I'm a biological female, and it would never occur to anyone that I was pregnant. I figure the first six months, everyone will just think I'm getting fat. And then I'll quit work for the last trimester. No one will know."

Darla and Eric had met at a transgendered event. They'd been together for five years, married for three.

"Were you married as man and woman, as Eric and Darla?" I asked. "Is that what shows up on your marriage license?"

"Yes," Darla answered.

"Please forgive my ignorance," I said, "but is that legal?"

"We think so, but we never really investigated it too much," Eric responded. "I changed my legal name to Eric, and Darla changed hers to Darla. So why would anyone pay any attention?"

"What about your sex life?" I asked.

"The testosterone has been great for my sex drive," said Eric, "but Darla hasn't had much desire as long as I've known her." She nodded in agreement. "That's okay. Our relationship isn't based on sex."

"I lost my erections as soon as I went on the estrogen," Darla added. "I get a good woody every now and again, but it's not too often, and not necessarily because I'm thinking about sex," she added.

"Can you ejaculate?" I asked Darla.

"It's been years," she replied, a bit glumly, I thought. "Will that affect my ability to have a baby?"

"It could," I answered carefully, "but I suspect that if you go off your hormones to make sperm, as we discussed before, your ability to have an ejaculation will likely come back too. It's all connected. One other option to consider instead of a vasectomy reversal is a simpler operation in which I can collect sperm from the testicles without putting the tubes back together again. Because there are so many fewer sperm, though, that procedure would commit the two of you to doing in vitro fertilization. Do you know what that is?"

"Yes," Eric answered. "That's where they put the sperm and eggs together in a dish in the laboratory, and the fertilized eggs then get put back inside my uterus a few days later."

"That's right," I said, impressed at the clarity of Eric's description. He was clearly knowledgeable about this topic, which made it all the more surprising that he seemed unaware of the fact that he would need to go off his hormone treatments before and after becoming pregnant.

"We're not interested in IVF," said Eric. "We want to have a baby naturally or not at all."

A couple of weeks later I received a phone call from Darla, with some follow-up questions. At the end of the call, she said that Eric was very concerned about going off his hormones. They hadn't decided what to do yet but were also looking into adoption. I never heard from them again. They wanted a child. Of this I had no doubt. However, it was even more important to them to each be able to remain the person they had struggled so long to become.

"I Never Felt Like a Boy"

Shortly after meeting Effie, as I was about to enter exam room #2 in my office, my secretary passed by me in the hallway, whispering, "You're going to love your next patient. She is soooo adorable." I glanced at the chart, knocked on the door, and entered.

There was Alicia, twelve years old, cute as a button, delicate, pretty face, brown hair parted on the side flowing down just below her shoulders, with a tiny braid of only a few strands of hair mixed in. I smiled, introduced myself, and held out my hand. She grabbed it uncertainly, as children often do, and then I shook hands with her father, Bill, standing next to her.

"I like your shoes," I said to Alicia, and she glanced down with pride at her clear plastic flip-flops with a white flower emerging between her big toe and the next.

"Thank you," she replied shyly.

"Why have you come to see me today?" I asked. Alicia looked toward her father, exchanging glances that suggested they'd been rehearsing this conversation.

"Dr. Spack said you could put that little pellet thingy in my arm that will help me with my hormones." Her eyes met mine for a moment, and then she glanced down again at her shoes.

"And tell me why you want help with your hormones, Alicia." She looked uncertain.

"Go on, tell the doctor," said Bill warmly. "We've been through this. It's all right."

Alicia hesitated, then raised her face bravely. "To make it easier for me to be a girl," she answered.

"That's right. Good job," said her father approvingly.

"How long have you been living as a girl?" I asked. "Dressing like a girl, for instance."

"I've been wearing dresses since I was nine, but before that I always wore clothes that were kinda in-between. I didn't feel right in boys' clothes since I was three. That was when I knew I was really a girl. Ever since I can remember, I never felt like a boy. Dr. Spack told me a lot of kids figure it out around that time." (Norman Spack, MD, of Children's Hospital Medical Center in Boston is a pioneer in helping youngsters with sexual identity issues, called gender dysphoria.)

I nodded. "How are things at school?" I asked.

Alicia raised her eyebrows as if this were a strange question. "School's great," she answered simply.

"I mean, does everyone at school treat you like a girl?"

"Oh yes," she said, nodding her head up and down.

"She goes to a great school," interjected Bill. "We've been very lucky. All the teachers, the school counselor, the kids, and even the other parents have been terrific."

I was glad to hear it. It is not unusual for children like Alicia to be exposed to a great deal of unpleasantness at school.

"Do you have any brothers and sisters?" I asked.

"Yes. Billy Jr. is fourteen."

"How are things with him?"

"Fine. He's into sports. He's okay with me."

Alicia was born a boy named Bruce. Very early on, he felt that something was terribly wrong, that a mistake had been made, since he felt certain in his heart of hearts that he was really a girl. For several years Alicia had been under the care of a psychologist, psychiatrist, and pediatrician. Now Alicia had come under the care of Dr. Spack, who had prepared Alicia for the hormonal treatment that would be required for her to live as a girl, and for the possibility of surgery later on. None of these professionals believed that Alicia was crazy or confused. On the contrary, the reports indicated that Alicia was psychologically healthy and well adjusted. As a girl. All of these professionals supported Alicia's decision to undergo hormone treatment.

Alicia had been referred to me so that I could place a small implant under her skin that slowly secretes a medication to suppress testosterone production from the testicles. Similar medications are available as injections, but those must be taken several times a year and are very expensive. The implant can last two years or longer in adolescents, resulting in fewer treatments and significantly lower cost.

In Alicia's case there was no time to lose in beginning treatment. Once puberty started, the marked rise in testosterone would cause irreversible changes in her body, changes that would forever mark her as a man. It is testosterone at the time of puberty in boys that causes definition and growth of muscles, stimulates facial hair to grow as a beard, and brings about enlargement of the larynx, which in turn deepens the voice and forms the Adam's apple. Preventing Alicia's pubertal rise in testosterone would ensure that her appearance would remain more delicate and feminine, far better than anything that could be achieved with makeup or plastic surgery once the testosterone-driven changes took place.

On examination, Alicia's penis was still the small appendage of a young boy, and her testicles were pea-sized. Puberty had not yet begun. However, a few dark hairs in the pubic region provided a telltale sign that it was not that far off.

Alicia's mother had died just six months earlier from breast cancer when she was only forty-one years old. Alicia's mom had been a tireless advocate for her. She believed what her child said when he insisted he had never felt like a boy. She had supported her son when he wanted to wear girls' clothing, and had watched him transform from an unhappy, anxious boy into a happy, carefree girl. Alicia's mom found sympathetic doctors and psychologists who helped the entire family find their way through the maze of resistance, criticism, prejudice, and lack of understanding they all encountered. At school she met with the teachers, principal, counselors. She normalized the experience with other parents and their kids, many of whom knew Alicia as Bruce from when the children were all much younger.

Now Alicia's mom was gone, and her dad had jumped in, doing his best to be as effective an advocate for Alicia as his wife had been. Alicia's wish to be able to feel "normal" as a female when her body was male was not a capricious fancy. It had been a several-year journey that had involved the entire family, challenging all of their emotional and financial resources.

I spoke with Alicia about the procedure, which would be done in the office under local anesthesia.

"Will it hurt?" asked Alicia.

"Not very much," I answered. "The numbing medicine will sting, like when you get a shot, but after that you shouldn't feel anything bad at all. The whole thing only takes a few minutes."

Alicia looked at her father anxiously.

"You can do this, honey," he said lovingly, his hand gently rubbing her back.

"Okay." Alicia turned her gaze back to me. "I'm ready," she said bravely.

Alicia's Procedure

Alicia lay on my exam table, her left arm outstretched but bent at the elbow. "As if you were hitchhiking," I instructed, positioning her arm as I wondered to myself if anyone under forty even knows what hitchhiking is anymore. Alicia glanced anxiously at her father, who was sitting by her right side, holding her hand. Every now and then she would scrunch her eyes shut, then open them widely as if mentally preparing herself for what was to come.

"Okay, this is the numbing medicine," I warned. "Ready?" Alicia nodded her head slightly. "You're going to feel it now," I said, and I punctured her skin, raising a small wheal where I would make the incision. "Count to twenty, slowly, and the stinging will be all over by then. Okay?"

Alicia let out a tiny squeal, then relaxed within a few seconds when she realized it didn't hurt very much at all.

"You're doing great," said Bill.

We chatted a little as I made a tiny horizontal incision, then inserted the two-inch-long spaghetti-like implant just under the skin. Two Steri-Strips brought the skin edges together, and I then covered all of it with a small bandage. "That's it," I said.

"Really?" Alicia asked. She smiled in relief at her father, who smiled broadly back at her, still holding her hand.

Alicia sat up, rubbed her arm, and felt for the implant.

"I can't feel it," she said. "Oh wait, there it is," she declared, running her finger across the skin. "Doesn't feel hardly like anything," she noted approvingly. I then explained to Alicia and Bill how to care for the wound, and we said our good-byes.

As they walked toward the door, I overheard Bill say to Alicia, "Mom would be so proud of you, honey."

"Can I tell her?" Alicia asked.

"Sure, honey. Go ahead."

Alicia turned her head upward, as baseball players do after they hit a home run. "Momma! I did it!" she exclaimed. Bill put his arm on Alicia's shoulders, and they walked out the door, a proud, loving father and his daughter.

The Transgender Issue

The transgender issue is complicated. A colleague asked why I wanted to get involved in "treating these adolescents who are just confused about their own sexuality." Yet after treating a fair number of these individuals, on the whole I have found these youngsters to be unusually grounded and mature for their age, and often very articulate about how they feel. In a couple of cases I was concerned about other issues at play, such as attention-seeking, and I declined to treat them, sending them back to their referring physician. Except for those rare exceptions, what has struck me about these kids is the similarity of their stories and their straightforwardness about what they want.

Most of us have never experienced a single doubt as to whether we are a boy or girl, man or woman. We may struggle with how *well* we fulfill some romantic notion of our own manliness or femininity, but the basic gender issue, "Am I a boy?" or "Am I a girl?" never comes into play. Imagine what it must be like for a child to struggle with this most basic identity issue of all. We are all familiar with the stories of gay individuals who struggled with declaring their "differentness" to the world. Imagine how much harder it must be for a pre-adolescent like Alicia to stand up to family, friends, teachers, and clergy and declare, "I may look like a boy (or girl), but this is not who I am."

These kids have my sympathy and admiration. By the time they have come to see me, all have experienced a measure of criticism, ridicule, and sideways glances that would be difficult for the most self-confident of adults to withstand gracefully. To me, the best explanation to account for that kind of inner strength is that these kids have a certainty about who they are and who they are not. They are as sure about their true psychical gender as I am about mine.

Is it biological, then? Can the brain be female when the body is male? Current science believes that the brain is imprinted as a male by two transient bursts of testosterone during fetal and neonatal life. If hormones are critical for the brain to become male, then perhaps some glitch in that early testosterone production (e.g., too little, too late) could account for the body developing as a male but not the mind. A deeper question is where our self-identification as male or female comes from, but hard answers to that question are difficult to come by.

An Uncomfortable Class

One day during medical school my renowned professor of reproductive biology, wearing his signature bow tie, shut off the lights
and flipped on the slide projector. The very first image made me
squirm. It was a photo of a woman. I think she had an attractive
face, but I couldn't say for sure, because my attention was focused
on the fact that she was quite naked, with large breasts and curvy
hips. Slides of several more naked women quickly followed, all
quite Marilyn Monroe–esque, with hourglass figures. Some of the
women had black rectangles superimposed over their eyes, providing a degree of anonymity; however, the photos did not appear
particularly medical.

It was a small, dark room, with only about fifteen to twenty
students, some of whom were women, and the projector's motor
made a whirring sound. It was an uncomfortable moment—should
we be looking at this kind of stuff in school? This was an early
class in the semester, so we hardly knew the professor. Was he
some kind of pervert? I looked around. Other students looked
uncomfortable too.

"Lovely, aren't they?" intoned the professor. "Some have been
Playboy centerfolds. However, it's time to snap out of your rever-
ies, especially the gentlemen!" he suddenly exclaimed in a louder,
more professorial voice. "These women have all been my patients,
and they all have the same condition. Anyone want to guess what
it is?"

No one said anything, but I saw my fellow classmates relax, as
did I. At least we were back into medical territory. "Here's a clue,"
he offered. "All of these women came to medical attention as young
women because they had never menstruated."

No one spoke up, and he showed a few more slides. "Here is a
photo of the external genitalia of one of them. And here is another,"
he said, advancing the slides. We saw what appeared to be normal
labial folds, a clitoris, the urethral opening for urine in the correct
location. All looked normal, not that any of us, male or female,

was a particular expert in female anatomy at that age, regardless of how some of the guys might describe themselves in public or over drinks. "Any guesses now regarding the diagnosis?" he asked the group. None came. We were dumbfounded and, speaking for myself, still more than a bit uncomfortable.

"What are the causes of amenorrhea?" he asked, using the medical term for the absence of menstrual cycles.

"Hormonal abnormalities" was one answer.

"Pituitary tumors" came another.

Now the class was engaged. Ovarian problems, uterine pathology, genetic abnormalities were all suggested. "Hysterectomy with bilateral salpingo-oopherectomy," one voice called out, referring to the surgical procedure in which the uterus, ovaries, and Fallopian tubes are all removed.

The professor nodded his head approvingly but gave away no hint whether any of us had hit on the correct answer. "Here are blood test results for one of these women." He showed a slide with test results on the screen for a minute and then advanced the slide. "And here are results for another of these women."

Most of the results were within the normal range; however, testosterone concentrations in both cases were many times higher than normal for women. For that matter, they were unusually high even for men.

"It's a testosterone-secreting tumor!" blurted out one student.

"Well, not exactly, but you're closer than you might think." He chuckled, pleased by our confusion. "And here," he continued, advancing through a few slides, "is an image of the surgical findings." The first image showed a normal opening to the vagina, but the vaginal canal itself was quite short. A slide of the inside of the pelvis taken during surgery was notable for what was *not* present. There was no uterus, no ovaries, no Fallopian tubes. Instead, we saw one gonad with a pearly white surface, deep in the pelvis on the right. A separate photo from the outside showed a pair of forceps pointing to a bulge within the left labium majorum, the outer "lips" surrounding the vagina.

These women were men. More precisely, these individuals were genetic males, with a normal male karyotype of 46XY, and a condition called testicular feminization. The two gonads were testicles. One had descended as far as it could, into the labial tissue because there was no scrotum, and the other simply hadn't descended. Unlike Effie, there was no uterus or similar structures to block the descent of the testicles. The uterus was absent because during development these individuals had presumably produced anti-Müllerian factor in the proper way at the proper time. This was why none of them had ever menstruated. So why did they look like women?

Their problem is a rare genetic mutation that makes the body unable to recognize testosterone. Hormones work by binding to a receptor, like a key fitting a lock, and the mutation caused the receptor to be defective. Testosterone levels were higher than normal for a woman because these individuals had normally functioning testicles, and testosterone levels were higher than normal for men because the regulatory system continually called for extra testosterone production since it mistakenly sensed there was none in the bloodstream.

These individuals are assumed to be female at birth, live as women, and pass through normal puberty as women. They come to medical attention as teenagers or young adults because they do not menstruate, and they cannot become pregnant. Otherwise, no one would ever know. The reason so many of them have lovely figures, with prominent breast development, is that they have high levels of estrogen, which is converted directly from testosterone. Experience from transgendered populations indicates that the best conditions for breast development occur when estrogen is high and testosterone is low. In these cases, the body detects no testosterone, so it behaves as if there were none. Popular rumor in medical circles has it that more than one well-known female actress, admired for her ample cleavage, has the condition of testicular feminization.

The incredible lesson about our sexual biology is that all men, at one point in their fetal development, have the capacity to be women. Moreover, the body is programmed to develop as a female unless it sees and recognizes specific biochemical signals, such as testosterone and anti-Müllerian factor, that tell it to develop as a male.

Where Does Sexual Orientation Fit In?

The discussion of gender gets even more complicated when we throw sexual orientation into the mix. A primary care physician from the student health services at a local university called me one day to ask if I would see a female student who complained of painful erections. A woman with painful erections? Sure.

Jayne came to see me the next day. She was twenty-four years old, attractive in a student-Bohemian way, with long, wavy chestnut hair to the middle of her back, wearing a white button-down blouse and fashionably torn jeans. She appeared totally at ease when I asked her to explain why she had come to see me. "Doctor, for the last six to eight months I get an unpleasant, painful feeling in my penis every time I get an erection. It's really put the kibosh on my sex life."

By now, you won't be surprised to learn that Jayne was born male and had chosen to live as a female at age twenty-one. Unlike Alicia, her hormonal treatment had begun after the onset of puberty and consisted primarily of high-dose estrogen, which stimulates breast development and suppresses testosterone. Jayne had undergone laser treatment to remove the hair follicles where her beard should have been, and she looked very much a woman despite the slight prominence of her Adam's apple.

I mentioned to Jayne that many men I see with very low or suppressed testosterone levels have a difficult time having any erections at all. Had she noticed something similar when she began hormone treatment?

"Well, since I started hormone treatment I almost never get morning erections anymore," she answered matter-of-factly. "Or erections from thinking about sex. I mainly get erections now when I'm dating someone."

"Do you tend to date men or women?" I asked.

"Oh, women!" she responded, as if there could be no question about it.

"And when you have sex, do you put your penis inside?"

"Well, I used to until I started having this pain!" Jayne laughed wryly.

Jayne had a condition of the penis called Peyronie's disease, in which scar tissue within the penis develops due to underlying inflammation. When the penis attempts to expand during erection, the scar tissue fails to stretch normally, and the penis curves, creating an unpleasant, pulling sensation. Jayne and I discussed possible treatments, including injections and surgery. However, Jayne was planning to surgically complete her gender transformation within the next few years, which would eliminate any penis problems altogether.

"I can deal with this," Jayne said. "I just wanted to make sure it wasn't anything more serious."

Here was an individual born as a man, who felt like a woman, and whose sexual interest was women. By changing her gender, but continuing to sleep with women, Jayne technically became gay in the process. Our overly rigid ideas of how we think about sex, sexual identity, and sexual orientation ("That's not right!" "There's too much permissiveness in society!" "Bad parenting!") crumble when confronted by a story like Jayne's.

So What Is a Man?

The stories in this chapter may be unusual, yet they bring this question into stark relief. Is a man defined by having a penis? No. Females exposed to high levels of androgens (molecules with testosterone-like properties) during fetal life often have a hyper-trophied clitoris that is hard to distinguish from a boy's penis.

How about testicles? No. Individuals with testicular feminization have testicles, yet these individuals live quite happily as women.

Do we define a man genetically, then, by the presence of a Y chromosome? This is the definition of a genetic male, but surely it is not enough, since there are cases where the Y chromosome is present, but key genes are missing or dysfunctional, leading to a female appearance.

High testosterone levels? If this were the sine qua non of being a man, what do we call individuals with advanced prostate cancer who undergo treatment to reduce their testosterone to zero? Are they no longer men? This can't possibly be the definition of a man.

If genes, hormones, and anatomy cannot define a man, what are we left with? A passion for the *Godfather* movies, gambling, and mixed martial arts?

It is none of these things and yet all of them. Before we can proceed to investigate the nature of men, sexuality, and relationships, we must acknowledge that the almost-universal assumption of men as creatures entirely distinct from women is false.

Part of the confusion is that sexuality is expressed on at least three levels: gender identity (Do I feel like a boy or a girl?), anatomic gender (Do I have the parts of a boy or a girl?), and sexual orientation (Do I like boys or girls—or both—sexually?). What is intriguing, if a bit mind-boggling, is that all three of these levels of sexuality are independent of each other. Jayne, for example, went from having sex with women as a straight man, to having sex with women as a gay woman.

In my mind, there are two additional considerations: one is hormonal. Claudia, the mother of the preschooler I mentioned, at the beginning of this chapter, had it largely right when she attributed much of the behavioral differences between boys and girls to testosterone, even though at the age of our children back then the concentrations of testosterone in the blood was identical in both sexes. Testosterone masculinizes babies in the womb and soon after. And the large difference in testosterone concentrations between the sexes as adults influences so much of the physical and mental differences that we recognize between men and women.

The final level is even more difficult to define. I believe it is a cocktail of psychology, free will, and spirit. It is about how men behave. In Yiddish, there is an expression, "He's a mensch," which translates literally to "He's a man" but means much more. There is no simple, one-word equivalent for *mensch* in English, but it is a term of approval, indicating a man of integrity and honor, someone we would be happy to be associated with. There is no requirement for a Y chromosome, male genitalia, or even testosterone to be a mensch. This last feature of masculinity, then, is about how men behave, the choices they make, the way they move through this world as individuals with free will.

If we are to begin to honestly attempt to understand men and their sexuality, we have to start with a broader concept of *maleness*. There can be no doubt that there are important differences between men and women. Conventional terminology labeling men and women as opposites, as in *opposite sex*, makes no sense once we recognize how much we share.

5. A PENIS BY ANY OTHER NAME

Women are from stars, men are from penis.

—Vanna Bonta, American writer

Luke Gets a Penis

One day when I was still working at the hospital I stepped into the reception area, where about a dozen men and women sat waiting for doctors from different specialties. I called out the name of the next patient on my list for the day. Luke stood up and walked into my exam room, looking pretty much like any young man I might encounter: sandy brown hair, brown full beard trimmed short, jeans, and a T-shirt that listed tour dates for Bruce Springsteen and his E Street Band. I noticed on his paperwork that he lived several hours away by car.

"I was hoping you could do an operation on me that I've been researching," Luke said. "I've asked around, and a plastic surgeon in my town knew someone in Boston, and he recommended you. That's why I've traveled to see you."

"Well, I'm flattered," I said. "What's the operation?"

"It's called metoidioplasty," replied Luke. "Are you familiar with it?"

"I'm afraid I've never heard of it. What kind of operation is it?"

"It's an operation to convert my clitoris into a penis." Luke then pulled out some photocopied papers and a magazine article, and placed them in front of me on my desk.

Luke was a biological female. He was married and worked as a swim coach for a small community high school. For the last four years, Luke had lived as a man, taking testosterone, which helped him grow a full beard and gave his muscles definition. Like Eric, Luke had undergone a mastectomy to remove his breast tissue. "I didn't really have that much up top before anyway," he said. Luke's wife, Amy, was a teacher in the same school.

I leafed through the material Luke had brought for me. The magazine was actually a low-budget newsletter titled *FTM*, which Luke informed me stood for *Female to Male*. The article described the operation in quite a bit of detail, as performed by a physician in Thailand.

"I've looked into all sorts of options," said Luke. "I don't want a neophallus." *Neophallus* is the term for a new penis (*neo* = new, *phallus* = phallus or penis) surgically constructed from muscle, fat, and skin taken from other parts of the body, sometimes the leg, sometimes the forearm, and occasionally the lower abdomen. "They usually look weird, and it's rare to have good sensation. There are so many problems with them too."

Luke was right. Although some of the ones I'd seen looked very good, they were never perfect, and usually these cases required additional procedures to correct and refine the original construction. And some of them come out looking more like a fat blob of skin and fat hanging down from the pubic region than anything one would call a penis. "The advantage of the operation I want you to do," Luke continued, "is that it leaves me with my own equipment. I know it can't be full adult size. I just want something of my own that feels like a penis."

I asked Luke to take a seat on the examining table, and he athletically hopped up. When he dropped his pants, there was a rubber model of a penis and scrotum sitting in his underwear. It fit against his body and filled out his underwear like a man. "I wear the same thing in my swim suit," he informed me.

"That's brave of you to be seen in public in just a bathing suit," I commented. "Do you wear one of those long, bulky swimsuits?"

"No. This is a swim team. I wear a little Speedo, like everyone else."

"No one ever questions whether you're a man?"

"I don't think people ever think about it. My beard grew in great. I don't think anyone would ever suspect that someone with a beard like mine could be a woman."

I examined Luke. He had normal female genitalia, with one difference. His clitoris was unusually prominent, several times the normal size. Under the influence of testosterone it had hypertrophied remarkably and sat like a mushroom cap above the vagina.

It is always such a strange experience for me to examine a transgendered individual. When the genitalia are exposed, even when I know to expect what I'll see, I feel a disconnect. Our brains are hardwired, it seems, to make clear-cut judgments—girl or boy. In clothes, and even apparently in a Speedo, Luke passed easily as a man.

When Luke had dressed, I told him I'd never done this operation and I would need to research it before deciding whether I could help him. Over the next few weeks we were in touch a couple of times by phone, and eventually I agreed to do it. I warned Luke that the nerves could be injured, leaving the new penis without sensation, and the blood supply could also be injured, causing tissue loss. Most important, I told Luke I didn't know how good this penis would look or how long it would be.

"Doctor, I understand. I just want to have something that feels like a penis. It doesn't much matter to me how big it is."

Two months later Luke arrived for surgery. He was given general anesthesia, and then his legs were placed in stirrups, just like a woman at the gynecologist's office, so that I could stand and

work right in front of him. The clitoris is really the female ana-
logue of the penis. Both penis and clitoris are called phallic structures. The fetal phallus develops into a penis in a little boy and
into a clitoris in a girl. They have the same nerve supply that
comes under the arch of the pubic bone, and the same blood supply. It was my first operation ever on a clitoris, but thanks to these
similarities, I was familiar with the basic anatomy.

One thing that is different, of course, is that the urethra, the
urine channel, is totally separate from the clitoris, whereas it is
an obvious and critical part of a boy's penis. During development
within the womb, the urethra in a baby boy is created along the
underside of the penis by an infolding of skin and tissue to create
a tube that extends from what would have been the urethral opening in a woman, underneath the pubic bone, to the tip of the penis.
In some boys the formation of this tube doesn't quite complete its
closure all the way out, resulting in the urethral opening occur-
ring somewhere along the underside of the penis. This is called
hypospadias. Boys with hypospadias urinate from the underside
of the penis, or have the opening moved to the tip with surgery.

Another obvious difference between the penis and clitoris is
size. The clitoris is usually no more than 1 to 1.5 centimeters in
diameter, roughly half an inch, whereas the glans penis (head of
the penis) at its broadest point is much larger, usually 3 to 5 centimeters when flaccid, and larger when erect. Luke's treatment with
testosterone had caused his clitoris to grow to 2 centimeters in
diameter, the thickness of a boy's penis.

The most fascinating thing about the anatomy of the clitoris
is that it is really, truly, a smaller version of the penis. There is a
glans, or head, just like a penis, with its own little hood, an equivalent of the male foreskin. There is also a shaft, with two erectile
chambers called corpora cavernosa (the Latin term for "cavernous
bodies"), lined by a sheath called the tunica albuginea. However,
the shaft is hidden inside, attached to the underside of the pubic
bones and covered from view by skin and tissue. The clitoris
appears to be a little button, but it's all there. My main task with

Luke was to free up the shaft of the clitoris so that the clitoris could hang down, just like a penis.

The challenge in that was to do it without injuring the nearby delicate nerves and blood vessels that feed it. After several hours of careful dissection, Luke had about 7 to 8 centimeters of penis hanging down, approximately three inches. I then mobilized flaps of skin to cover the shaft. Luke now had a dangling penis. It was skinny, but its length was reasonable. I thought it looked very good.

During my rounds that evening I sat at Luke's bedside, and he told me how lucky he felt to have his wife, Amy. Amy had seen him through all his life and body changes, first when he wanted to go on hormones and dress like a man, and then when he decided to have this surgery.

"You and Amy were both female when you first got together, right?" I asked.

Luke nodded.

"Are you legally married?"

He smiled and nodded yes.

"And when the two of you were both female, did you consider yourself a lesbian?"

"Never," replied Luke, quietly but firmly. "I've always considered myself a man. Even when I looked female, I thought of myself as having a heterosexual relationship with Amy. It's like they say, I had always felt like a man trapped in a woman's body. And with Amy, I've always been the man, even before I went on hormones."

"What about Amy?" I asked. "Did she consider herself gay, or lesbian, when the two of you began dating?"

"Amy had never been with a woman before she met me," answered Luke. "We joke that she's still never been with one! I don't really know what Amy thought about it all. This is by far the best relationship of my life, and I'd like to think it's been pretty good for Amy too, even though it's been a bit unusual. I don't know what to do with categories like gay, lesbian, straight. They don't seem to apply very easily to me. Or Amy, for that matter. In the end, we're just people."

Luke returned to see me four months later. When I asked to examine him, he proudly dropped his pants and shorts. The rubber model of penis and scrotum was gone. Instead he had a penis hanging down.

"Does it get hard?" I asked.

"It gets fatter when I'm excited, but not really erect. That doesn't matter, though. I didn't expect that. The important thing is that I finally feel complete. And I no longer need to stuff my Speedos at the pool!"

Rebuilding a Penis

Donald was a thirty-two-year-old man who also wanted a penis, but his story was quite different from Luke's. Donald became psychotic and was hospitalized at a psychiatric hospital in the Boston area and placed on a locked ward. He escaped and somehow made his way to Cleveland, where he was picked up for unruly conduct by the police, who assumed he was drunk. In his jail cell, Donald got hold of a shard of glass, cut off his penis and scrotum, and flushed them down the toilet.

It had been three years since that incident when I met Donald. He had been on his medications and was doing very well, with no relapses. He held a clerical job at one of the local hospitals and lived at a monitored residential home.

A year earlier, a well-known plastic surgeon decided Donald seemed stable enough, and he operated to create a neophallus, using skin and muscle from the left forearm. He rolled the tissue into a cylinder and then connected the nerves and blood vessels from the stump of the penis (there was about an inch left) to appropriate nerves and vessels from the forearm graft. Amazingly, Donald's new rolled sausage of a penis took hold and survived. It even had sensation. But it had no ability to become erect.

Recently, Donald had started dating a woman named Celia, and he wanted his penis to work the way his old one did. So the plastic surgeon referred him to me. Donald seemed reasonably well adjusted when I met him in the exam room. His face didn't show much expression, and his mood appeared flat. Yet he spoke intelligently about his situation, his work, and his girlfriend. "I want to be able to have sex with my girlfriend," he said simply, explaining why he'd come to see me.

"What do you do now for sex?" I asked.

"We play around," he answered. "I have good feeling at the base, where my original penis was. Celia gets me off by rubbing down there. And I can get her off too, with my hand or mouth. But we both want to be able to have sex like regular people."

Undressed, Donald had a generous-sized neophallus. It looked pretty good, but no one would mistake it for a real penis. There was no head, although the plastic surgeon had created a raised circle of skin to try to reproduce the corona, or crown at the head of the penis. "My plastic surgeon says he has a new way of doing that," Donald offered. "He says we can try it again later."

"From where do you urinate?" I asked, not seeing a hole in the neophallus.

Donald lifted up the penis to show me. "Under here," he said. And there was the urethral opening, well below the stump of his original penis. The anatomy was really quite similar to that of Luke's once he'd had his operation—penis above, urinary opening below it.

"Do you have feeling in the new portion of the penis?" I asked.

"Uh, yeah. There's some feeling," he replied.

I checked Donald's sensation, lightly touching the top of the penis with my gloved finger. "Can you feel that?" I asked.

"No." Donald had better sensation on the left side and the underside.

I grasped a fold of skin and pinched it. "Can you feel this?" I asked.

"Yeah, I can tell you're there," he answered calmly. If Donald had had normal sensation, he would have jumped from pain.

After speaking with Donald's plastic surgeon, I agreed to go ahead and I scheduled surgery to place a penile implant in Donald's neophallus.

In the operating room I created a single chamber for the implant cylinder out of an artificial tube graft designed to replace diseased arteries. This tube would serve as Donald's new tunica albuginea, the sheath of the normal corpus cavernosum. I placed the graft into the neophallus and then opened one of the original corpora cavernosa from the stump of Donald's own penis. I dilated this area and placed the rear portion of the implant cylinder into his own tissues and the front part of the cylinder into the tube graft within the neophallus. Although penile implants come with two cylinders, one for each of the two corpora cavernosa, Donald's neophallus only had enough room for one. I then placed the pump into the small amount of scrotal skin that remained. Fortunately, Donald hadn't cut all of this off.

I sutured everything closed and gave the pump a few squeezes. Up rose the penis. It wasn't quite as firm as with two cylinders, but it did the job.

I saw Donald for follow-ups at one week and six weeks. He seemed excited. Celia came into the room with us at the second visit. I taught them both how to inflate and deflate the implant.

"This is so exciting!" Celia said, watching the penis go up and down.

"We're going to have fun with this new toy!" Donald winked at me.

Donald didn't keep any of his next appointments with me, but I ran into him by accident on a street near the hospital where he worked.

"How is everything working out from the surgery?" I asked.

"It's good, Doc. Celia is happy, and that's the important thing."

"Are you able to put it inside?"

"Yeah. That's why she's happy."

"*You* don't sound quite as happy," I noted.

"No, no. It's fine. It really is." I looked at him wonderingly. "The problem," he continued, "is that I can't come when I'm inside her. I don't have enough feeling."

"So what do you do?"

"When Celia has had enough, I pull out and she makes me come by stroking my stump, the way she used to. It's fine, Doc. You did a good job," he said, as if he were trying to reassure me.

A few years later I ran into Donald again. "Everything okay?" I asked.

"Still ticking like a Timex," he said.

"And how are things with Celia?"

"Oh, Celia and I broke up a long time ago." I must have looked concerned, because Donald seemed to want to cheer me up. "It's okay, Doc. I'm seeing somebody new. She's great. Listen, I've got to run. I'm late for an appointment with my shrink. See ya around," he said, as he marched away.

When I was younger, I lived in a world of certainty. I fit the mold of what other physicians said about surgeons: "Occasionally wrong, but never in doubt." My friends and I labeled actions, and people, as *cool* or *uncool*. Anything that fell outside the narrow bounds of our worldview of correctness was prey for ridicule. It pains me now to admit it, but back in the sleep-deprived, dehumanizing days of my surgical residency, my fellow residents and I would label patients *citizens* or *crazies* (or worse), based on snap judgments from dress, speech, grooming.

Once I started seeing my own patients it didn't take long for me to realize that life is more complicated. People's lives are full of challenges. What did I know about any of it?

In my first year as an attending physician, I treated a man in his early sixties with an aggressive bladder cancer. His only hope was to have his bladder removed, but at surgery, I found the tumor had spread everywhere. I went to speak to his wife, waiting for me in her husband's hospital room, and informed her of the grim prognosis.

"No!" she gasped, and grabbed my hand. "Doctor, what am I going to do without him?" she asked plaintively, her voice breaking, tears running down her cheeks.

I had no answer. I was uncomfortable and wanted to leave. I told myself I had performed my professional duty by informing her of the surgical findings, but she held me tightly by my hand, even as she sat down in her chair, and I had no choice but to sit next to her and experience her grief. Sitting with her, I realized I was a child when it came to the raw realities of life, and my judgments were nothing more than armor protecting me from the gritty emotions and uncertainties of life, allowing me to work emotionally detached from those who entrusted me with their bodies and health.

In the Sunday newspaper comics the other day an older man says to his grandson after a stranger was gruff with them, "Don't take it personally. Every person you meet is battling *something*, even though it may not be obvious to us what they're battling." How true.

I can't possibly know what it is like to be a child feeling with certainty that there is something terribly wrong with my body. The mother of a twelve-year-old girl transitioning to be a boy told me, "Livia was just six years old when she said to me, 'Mommy, what do you do when God has made a mistake?'" The least I can do is respect the fact that people live their own lives, with their own special stresses and struggles.

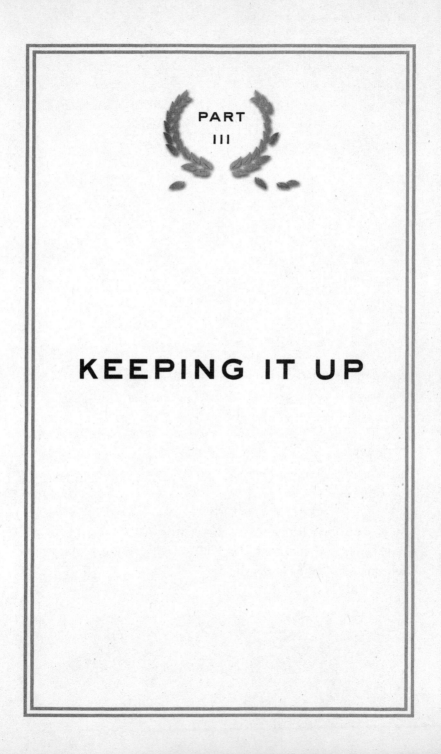

PART
III

KEEPING IT UP

6. BETTER LIVING THROUGH PHARMACOLOGY

*Doctors pour drugs of which they know little, to cure
diseases of which they know less, into patients of whom
they know nothing.*

—MOLIÈRE (1622–73), French dramatist

Philip was a retired, distinguished newscaster who had come
to see me. I had seen him many times on the television in
the past. Now, at eighty-two, he looked great: tall, erect posture,
handsome, full head of white hair. And he had a killer dry wit.

"My wife died three years ago after a long battle with breast
cancer," he said. "I wasn't planning on dating again, but a couple of
months ago my daughter decided it was time for me get back out
there. She introduced me to Anne, the mother of her friend, who
had lost her husband a few years ago. We all went out to dinner
together, the four of us, and I found myself looking over at Anne
a lot.

"We went on a few more dates—without our daughters—and
she's turned out to be a great lady. But I feel like I'm robbing the
cradle," he said with an impish gleam in his eyes.

"How old is she?" I asked.

"Seventy-three. Almost ten years younger than me—can you

imagine? I tease her that when I was in high school she was just learning how to spell her name." Badda bing.

"So how can I help you?" I asked, smiling.

"Well, Anne enjoys sex a lot, and my penis doesn't work that well anymore."

After an examination and a review of Philip's medical history and test results, I gave him a couple of samples of Cialis to try. They come in a brightly colored box, roughly the size of a package of cigarettes, with the trade name emblazoned on the front. We walked out into the hallway together, and I noticed that Philip was holding the Cialis samples in his hands, in plain view, rather than tucking them into his pocket as most men do.

"Philip, would you like me to get you a bag for the pills so that no one sees you have them?"

"Are you kidding?" he exclaimed. "I want *everyone* to see what I've got!"

It was an early fall barbecue at my home with my office staff. Several of them have young children, and the topic of conversation turned to how early in life male sexuality begins. Oscar, the father of a two-year-old boy, remarked, "I can't believe that a two-year-old gets erections. I didn't know that until I had Connor. Half the time when I change his diaper, there it is, standing up."

"I know!" chimed in Kai, the mother of a five-year-old. "Troy came into the living room the other day straight from the bathroom. His pants and underpants were off, and there he was pulling at his thing. 'Stop pulling at it,' I told him. He just thought it was funny. He's always touching it."

"Listen to this," said Val, the mother of an autistic twelve-year-old boy who has been mainstreamed into school. "Jimmy hasn't even hit puberty yet. Last week I went into his room to wake him up for school, and I noticed he had this strange smile on his face. I was about to wake him up, and then I saw he had a little tent pole lifting up the sheets." There was some chuckling at this common male experience happening to a child that many of us had known since he was a baby. "He seemed so happy," continued Val. "I decided to let him sleep for a few more minutes."

We are sexual creatures from our earliest days until we die. There is just no getting away from it.

Enter: Masters and Johnson

It is remarkable how much the world of human sexuality has changed within my professional lifetime. For men, there have been two major upheavals, revolutions actually, during that time, and a third is taking place right now. I have been fortunate to have been present at the front lines for these incredible changes, participating as best I could, learning from the world's masters, contributing where I could to the forum of ideas, and doing my best to provide my own patients with the best and most up-to-date treatments.

It will come as no surprise to most readers that one of these revolutions was the introduction of Viagra as an oral treatment for ED in 1998, and the soon-to-follow appearance of its brethren Cialis and Levitra. The newest revolution is the recognition of the importance of testosterone in the health and sexuality of men as well as women, which I will discuss in more depth in chapter 10. However, a change arguably even more profound than these occurred as a consequence of a number of events in the early 1980s. These events not only altered how we treat men with sexual issues but also changed our basic view of men in general.

I was fourteen years old in May 1970 and hungry to learn whatever I could about the mysterious world of sex when a copy of *Time* magazine arrived at our home with a cover story about William Masters, MD, his assistant, Virginia Johnson, and their work on human sexuality. It was eye-opening. Not just to me but to an entire generation. It is difficult for young men and women of today to imagine what it was like when there were only three network channels on television, no Internet, and fewer than half a dozen general-interest magazines. There was a limit to the sources of our information, and thus each one played a much larger role in informing us than the cacophony of competing media/Internet sites of today. *Time* magazine was one of those few sources, and the impact of any cover story in that magazine was big. A cover story about sex was *huge*.

Dr. Masters was a St. Louis gynecologist who set out to scientifically investigate what the human sexual response looked like. He hired Mrs. Johnson as his research assistant (and later married her after they each divorced their original spouses) because he felt it would be helpful for the women being studied to interact with a woman instead of a man. As they moved from pure investigation of sexuality into the arena of therapy for sexual issues, Masters and Johnson used almost exclusively two-person, male-female teams as models so that the men and women they were studying could relate to someone of their own sex. They used themselves and their own sexual relationship as models in their research as well.

The *Time* cover story coincided with publication of their second blockbuster book, *Human Sexual Inadequacy*, which described a variety of sexual problems for men and women, and reported their attempts to treat them. However, Masters and Johnson were already widely known for their first book, *Human Sexual Response*, published in 1966, which provided obsessively detailed information on what actually happens during sex. Amazingly, Masters and Johnson, as well as their assistants, would be in the same room as couples having sex, watching, taking notes, recording. Many, if not most, of the couples being observed and studied included at least one prostitute, male or female, which perhaps explains their ability to participate in a clinical setting. Determined and ever-resourceful, Masters and Johnson even designed a clear plastic dildo with a camera attached so that they could document what happened inside the vagina during simulated sex, making observations on lubrication and other physiological responses. The technical language they used didn't stop the book from gaining both notoriety and popularity.

It is hard to overstate the importance of Masters and Johnson to the zeitgeist of the time. The only comparable figure in the field of human sexuality was Alfred Kinsey; however, his primary contribution had been extensive surveys of sexual *behavior* in the 1940s and 1950s rather than in-depth observations about the biology of sex. The timing was crucial too. The late 1960s and early 1970s were a time of Vietnam war protests, hippies, Woodstock, the introduction of the Pill (oral contraceptive), and the birth of the "free sex" era. Much of the United States was undergoing a period of sexual liberation, leaving behind prudish attitudes from the stuffy 1950s and early 1960s. Masters and Johnson were the Rock Stars of Sex. Their pronouncements were the stuff of certainty.

This is what I, along with a huge swath of the reading public, learned about sexuality from the *Time* cover story of Masters and Johnson: penis size has little to do with sexual effectiveness; there is no physiologic difference between a clitoral and vaginal orgasm; masturbation is not harmful; intercourse can take place safely throughout pregnancy unless there are specific problems such as bleeding or pain; and communication is the key to a satisfying sexual relationship. As an amateur historian of sexual medicine, it is fascinating for me to go back today and read contemporaneous descriptions of their work. What is striking is that despite the boldness of bringing these accurate and useful ideas into the public arena, none of these ideas became associated with Masters and Johnson. No, the single most important and enduring piece of information attributed to Masters and Johnson was something else entirely, and their assertion influenced an entire generation of men and women; they concluded that the vast majority of men with impotence had a psychological basis for their sexual inadequacy.

Today, few if any educated persons who came of age after the early 1980s have even heard of Masters and Johnson. There can be many reasons why prominent historical figures lose their purchase on our consciousness, but in my opinion the most important one in this case is simple: they were wrong. Totally, absolutely wrong. However, it took approximately twenty years to figure that out. In the meantime, the public and medical world operated with the certainty that their conclusions were true. The impact was powerful and remarkably negative.

I have argued here that we still know precious little about sexuality in ways that matter, but by comparison with the 1960s, 1970s, and most of the 1980s, we are all savants. Imagine being a man with ED living in a time when no one discussed sex with anyone else, there was no information about how common the condition was, everyone seemed to be having such a good time with their sexual "liberation," and everyone believed that impotence was psychological. Men with ED who had always considered themselves sane, grounded, balanced were taught to believe that they were no longer psychologically sound. Something was wrong with them. They began to believe they had a tragic flaw, a weakness of spirit, will, determination. Or worse.

When I began my practice in 1988 at the end of the Masters and Johnson era, as I like to think of it, things were shifting within scientific circles as evidence began to show that ED was common and usually physical in nature. That shift took time to take root in the public consciousness, and for several years I saw one man after another who felt confused, diminished by what he perceived as a failure of his masculinity.

"I don't understand it, Doctor," said Jonathan, a married fifty-two-year-old social worker with diabetes and hypertension who had developed progressive difficulties with erection over the last two years. "I've spent my career helping others with emotional and psychological problems, and thought I'd worked through my own 'stuff' a long time ago. I feel horrible, for my wife, and for myself too, that I'd been completely unaware that one day a deep psychological issue of mine would kick me in the teeth like this. I've been seeing a psychiatrist for a few months now and trying to figure out what happened in my past that has made me become such a poor excuse for a man." After a few questions it was clear that Jonathan had garden-variety ED on a physical basis, common among diabetics and men with hypertension. Yet Jonathan, along with so many men like him at that time, was prepared to believe he had failed in a way that was psychological and under his control.

It is interesting to look at the term *sexual inadequacy*, which was used a lot during the Masters and Johnson era and was even incorporated in the title of their second book. They employed it to describe all sorts of sexual problems, including failure of women to reach orgasm, lack of sexual interest, and also erection problems. I suppose *adequacy* might be a reasonable term for a scientific inquiry, but I simply cringe at the thought of men and women already shamed by having these problems, hearing or reading that they are "inadequate." These folks felt inadequate already. To have their own, personal fears substantiated in negative language by the medical community, to be told their problems came from their own psychological deficiencies, must have been humiliating and depressing.

Another problematic term was *impotence*. *Impotence* is the traditional term for erection problems, but it also means weak, powerless, ineffectual. It is certainly true that men with impotence do feel that way, but is it really necessary to rub it in? Thankfully, in 1992 the U.S. National Institutes of Health convened a consensus conference on impotence, and one of its primary recommendations was to replace the term *impotence* with *erectile dysfunction*, which we now often refer to as *ED*. Just as an individual with a poorly functioning kidney is said to have renal dysfunction, and liver disease is called hepatic dysfunction, so now a man with a penis that doesn't work properly is said to have erectile dysfunction.

In the United States today the term *impotence* has fallen out of favor. Curiously, the term is still in use in England. In 1999 I wrote a review article for the respected journal the *Lancet*. My original title was "Erectile Dysfunction in Men." The London-based editors changed it to "Male Impotence." Ah, well. Perhaps they'll come around someday too.

Maybe It's Not All in Your Mind

I chuckle to myself when I think back to the beginning of my career. Not so much because my colleagues and I were naive (although we were) but more because of how things have changed so dramatically. I believe that psychotherapy can be enormously helpful for men and women with psychological issues, and over the years I have referred a large number of men and their partners to therapists, with whom I have had strong and productive relationships. However, it is a totally different story when a part of a man's body stops working well and the world has conspired to tell him it is all in his head.

One of the difficulties of practicing psychology is that it is a "soft science." There is no blood test or objective measurement one can make to determine the exact cause of a person's psychological problem. When I started in the field, there was an endless set of possible psychological causes for ED, and many of them were often believed to have occurred in childhood: a bad relationship with one's mother or father as a child, sleeping in the same bed as one's parent, bed-wetting, walking in on one's parents (or anyone else) having sex, an overbearing stepfather, a distant mother, a successful older sibling, a successful younger sibling, physical abuse, corporal punishment, anxiety, lack of interest, a bad sexual experience in the past, fear of commitment, fear of intimacy, fear of the vagina. The list went on and on. The literature, especially the psychiatric literature, was full of case reports of new and exotic psychological explanations for impotence.

At that time the emphasis in the field of psychiatry was talk therapy. Today, that almost seems quaint when antidepressants are so freely prescribed, and visits to the psychiatrist take fifteen minutes of discussing medication dosage and side effects. When I was in medical school and residency, any man with impotence who desired treatment would be referred to a shrink. The solution to ED, or impotence as it was still called, was believed to lie in identifying the source of the psychological conflict or injury, and once identified, resolving it through the process of psychotherapy.

By the early to mid-1980s, a number of events had shown the truth that the vast majority of cases were physical, not psychological. It took some time for this truth to permeate the medical system and even longer to become accepted among the general population, but after that, it was impossible to deny its obviousness. Within a few short years, a cultural concept that had informed more than a generation of clinicians and the public had been shown to be false.

Even during the Masters and Johnson era it was well known that some serious medical conditions could cause physical impotence. These included advanced neurological conditions and severe arterial disease. A number of treatments had been attempted for these men, including surgery to bypass blocked arteries, as well as the penile implant (described in more detail in chapter 9), which was revamped in 1973 and was becoming ever more useful. However, there was no effective pharmacological treatment for ED. A chemical called yohimbine, derived from the plant *Pausinystalia yohimbe*, had been manufactured into pill form and had been touted for years as an aphrodisiac and sexual stimulant, and was prescribed for some men with ED, but it didn't really work.

Although it was understood for centuries that the two paired cylinders within the penis called the corpora cavernosa were, when filled with trapped blood, responsible for the rigidity of an erection, the key question that hadn't yet been answered in the 1980s was how exactly the blood became trapped within the penis in the first place.

To develop and maintain enough rigidity to go inside the vagina, the penis requires a mechanism to trap the additional blood that is released in the initial stage of an erection. Otherwise, the increased blood flow stemming from sexual arousal would just flow into the penis and flow out through the veins, making the penis full, or tumescent as we like to say in the business, but never hard. There is no other structure in the body with a venous draining system that allows blood to leave regularly at one time and then changes to a system where the blood is trapped at high pressures.

One older theory to explain this venous trapping of blood was based on microscopic analysis of veins on the surface of the tunica albuginea, the tough fibrous sheath encircling the corpora cavernosa. Published photomicrographs of those veins showed areas of thickening that appeared different from other veins in the body, and in the accompanying article the authors proposed that these thickened areas, called pollsters, acted as gates that could be open or close off the venous outflow depending on whether or not the penis was erect or flaccid. But there was no explanation for how the pollsters would become activated.

A competing theory was that a more superficial layer of tissue called Buck's fascia compressed the veins and prevented the venous outflow as the corpora cavernosa swelled with the added inflow of arousal and the outer tunica albuginea pushed against Buck's fascia. Laboratory experiments with animals failed to support either theory.

As the study of the male erection developed, scientists began to pay attention to the corpora cavernosa themselves. The inside of the corpora cavernosa is like a sponge, with cavernous spaces lined with smooth muscle. Muscle contracts and relaxes; this action is critical for the regulation of the arterial system that brings blood to all the tissues in the body. It seemed logical that the presence of muscle in the corpora cavernosa, vascular structures after all, was responsible for the on-off erection mechanism that could trap blood within the penis.

Keep Your Pants On!

Advances in medicine and science do not necessarily move forward in a series of considered steps, with each study adding to our knowledge incrementally. More often than not, science, like evolution, is propelled by major disruptions. In the world of male sexuality, that disruption was caused by an eccentric British neurophysiologist named Giles Brindley, who in 1983 gave a lecture that would change the field forever. Over the years I've asked several of my colleagues who attended what it was like, and they all smile and shake their heads in wonder.

Recently, at a meeting of the Sexual Medicine Society of North America (yes, such a society really does exist!), I sat down with Irwin Goldstein, MD, accompanied by his wife, Sue, to talk about the shift from the Masters and Johnson psychological model of erections and ED to the physical model that followed. Irwin has been, in my opinion, the single most important figure in the world of sexual medicine over the last thirty years. During that period, wherever and whenever there was something important happening in the field, Irwin was there, often as the leading figure. A high-energy, enthusiastic, irrepressibly cheerful man, Irwin trained dozens of individuals who went on to achieve their own academic prominence. Several years ago he moved to San Diego, where he established the first department of sexual medicine in the country at Alvarado Hospital Medical Center.

"Before Giles Brindley," explained Irwin, "we knew erection must be controlled somehow by smooth muscle. But we didn't know whether smooth muscle in the penis caused erections by contracting or relaxing. Actually, the scientific community at the time was divided into two camps: 'the vascular relaxation camp' and 'the vascular contraction camp.' After Brindley, there was no more discussion. It was settled."

"Were you there?" I asked.

"Of course," he replied. "I was one of the speakers on the same program."

"What happened?"

"It was incredible. It was 1983, in Las Vegas, at the annual meeting of the AUA [American Urological Association]. There was a specialty program for the Urodynamics Society. It was organized by Jacques Susset from Rhode Island . . . a neuro-urologist who was becoming interested in the neurology of erection. It was a big meeting with approximately three hundred to four hundred people in the audience."

"Some of the men were in tuxedoes," added Sue. "There were a lot of wives there too, some in gowns, because folks were planning on going out for dinner after the program."

"So," continued Irwin, "I'm arranging my slides before my talk at the table where the audiovisual guys sit, I'm dressed in a suit and tie, and this guy I'd never seen before, who turns out to be Giles Brindley, is arranging his slides too. Except that he's dressed in this athletic gear, you know, a jogging suit, one of those matching top and bottom get-ups with a zipper down the front. I thought it was very strange. Right before the program was about to begin I went into the bathroom, and there he was too.

"Brindley gets up for his lecture, still wearing the track suit, and starts showing photos of human penises at various stages of erection. It's all very scientific, with a grid behind the penis so that one can see the angle of the erection. He's talking about the effects of different medications on human erection. It was fascinating. It was the first talk on pharmacologic treatment of erections that I can recall. We had yohimbine, but that didn't really work. Brindley was injecting medicine, phenoxybenzamine, into the corpora cavernosa and achieving full erections.

"Then he informs the audience that the photographs are of his own penis! The audience starts laughing and giggling. Finally, he says, 'Oh hell,' or whatever the British equivalent is, and says, 'I guess I need to demonstrate this for you.' He goes on to say something like, 'Twenty minutes ago I injected my right corpus cavernosum with such-and-such milligrams of phenoxybenzamine, a medication that causes smooth muscle relaxation, and this is the result.' He drops his jogging pants, and he's got a full erection. At which point I realized that when I'd seen him in the toilet, he'd gone in there to inject himself!

"People were going crazy. There was a lot of laughter, and I think he was concerned they were laughing at him, because he seemed to get a bit angry. So he stepped into the audience, down the aisle with his pants still down at his knees, asking people to feel his erection. I think he wanted to prove it wasn't a penile prosthesis. I'm not sure that anyone actually felt it.

"There were two speakers on the program after him, including the moderator, Emil Tanagho, who was a huge figure in urology. No one listened to them. Everyone was still talking about Brindley's presentation. It was the most important lecture in the history of the AUA, and it immediately changed our medical practice. Within a week of getting home I put patients on injections. And it solved once and for all the questions about how erection occurred."

Brindley was not the first to inject medicine into a penis to help with erections. In France, the cardiovascular surgeon Ronald Virag, MD, injected the smooth muscle relaxant papaverine into a major artery in the pelvis when it went into spasm, and noted that the patient developed an erection even while asleep on the table. Chronologically, Virag gets credit for being first to hit upon the idea that medications injected into the penis that cause vessels to expand could cause an erection. In 1982 he published a letter in the *Lancet* describing the erection that occurred in men upon injection of papaverine.

When I asked Irwin Goldstein why Brindley's lecture had such an impact when Virag had already published his work the previous year, he replied, "There wasn't that much awareness yet of Virag's work. He wrote it up as a brief letter, and urologists didn't routinely read the *Lancet*. Brindley? Everyone who was at that lecture knew he had seen the future of the field, right then and there."

Brindley is a fascinating character. As a neurophysiologist (he is not a medical doctor) working at the London Hospital and the University of London, he had a track record of self-experimentation that I came across on more than one occasion during my investigation of reproductive issues. One of Brindley's papers reported on his research into the internal temperature of the scrotum. The reason the testicles lie outside the main part of the body, in the scrotum, is that they are extremely sensitive to high temperature. Indeed, core body temperature, ninety-eight degrees Fahrenheit, or thirty-seven degrees Celsius, is lethal for developing sperm cells. To assess how scrotal temperature varies over the course of the day and is influenced by clothing and by various positions, such as sitting and lying, Brindley came up with the clever idea of implanting a special thermometer within the scrotum for twenty-four hours. At this point the reader will not be surprised to learn that the subject for this experiment was Brindley himself. He cut into his own scrotum with a scalpel, implanted the device, and removed it the following day, his mission accomplished and his data collected.

Many paraplegics are unable to ejaculate due to their spinal cord injuries, rendering them infertile. Borrowing from breeding experience in animals, Brindley experimented with an electric probe inserted into the human rectum that might be able to stimulate an ejaculation for paraplegics and other men who were unable to do so on their own. Of course he was his own subject. In a 1981 scientific article, he described the effect of various voltages and amplitudes, and what sensations he experienced as the probe was rotated this way and that. He had to stop without successfully achieving an ejaculation when the voltage became too painful. In paraplegics, however, who lack normal sensation in the rectum and pelvis, he was able to achieve ejaculation at power settings several-fold higher than what he'd been able to tolerate himself.

I was intrigued. Around 1990 I contacted Professor Brindley to see if I could purchase an electro-stimulating device from him, since there was no commercially available equipment for this in the United States at the time. After some correspondence back and forth, I received it. The electrical box itself was simple—inelegant yet functional. The interesting part, though, was the electrical probe. It was a plastic, relatively narrow mound, designed to fit over one's index finger, and tapered at the tip where it would be inserted into the rectum. It was constructed of an off-white soft plastic material that felt rubbery. The surface was totally irregular, as if someone had whittled down a block of soap. A member of the hospital electrical department came to look it over, checked it out, and gave his approval. It looked homemade, because it was, yet the device was electrically sound and it worked flawlessly in many of my patients. Today we have other ways to help these men fertilize their partners without ejaculation, for instance, by harvesting sperm from the testicles, but at the time Brindley's electroejaculator was ingenious and the only thing we had.

The work of Brindley and Virag had an immediate and far-reaching effect. Not only was there now an effective medical treatment for ED, but the understanding of how erections worked had been catapulted forward. Techniques were rapidly developed based on the medications used by Brindley and Virag to study men with ED and compare them to men with normal erectile function. The first to be employed with any regularity was papaverine, often combined with another medication called phentolamine, which enhanced its efficacy. The next one used, and the only one approved so far by the FDA specifically for the treatment of ED, is called alprostadil, or prostaglandin E1.

The beauty of injections was that they required no arousal at all. The medicine, in humans or in animals, essentially flipped the switch biologically within the penis to "on." Finally, we had a way to really study the human penis within a laboratory setting. We learned how erections worked, and how they failed. A standard test dose of one of these vasoactive medications injected into the penis created firm, long-lasting erections in a man with intact plumbing within his corpora cavernosa, sometimes lasting several hours. If a man had significant vascular problems within the erectile chambers, injections led only to a soft or transient erection. Poor responses could still usually be overcome with stronger doses of medication, and not infrequently clinicians would combine all three of the most commonly used medications—papaverine, phentolamine, and alprostadil—in a solution called trimix, which was the most potent of all.

One of the first ideological casualties of this new wave of excitement was the Masters and Johnson rubric that ED was largely psychological. With rare exceptions, if a man was in a stable, relatively healthy relationship and his erections had declined progressively over a year or two or more, he was almost certain to have a suboptimal response to a test injection. Neither a failure of will nor an unrecognized emotional trauma as a child led to the man's weak erections as a grown-up. What he had was a physical problem within the penis. These injections were critical in turning the old "truth" about impotence on its head. Instead of 80 percent of impotent men having a psychological cause for their problem and 20 percent a physical cause, the new evidence indicated that the reverse was true: 80 percent of men who complained of weak erections had a physical cause for it, and perhaps 20 percent had a psychological cause.

The Singing Penis

In 1989 I read an article in the *Journal of Urology* by a group of Danish physicians who had found that one could measure electrical activity in the human penis, and this activity changed between the flaccid and erect state. They had placed electrodes into the penises of six normal men. One additional man—with diabetes and ED—had been included as a pathological control. Since smooth muscle relaxation was now known to control the process of erection, and muscular activity was associated with electrical currents that could be measured, this made perfect sense. I decided I wanted to look into this as a possible diagnostic test for men with ED.

In my clinic I borrowed a simple device from a neurology colleague that could measure electrical activity in muscles, and tried it in a few patients when flaccid and then after penile injections. I couldn't detect any signal at all. This was disappointing. I then contacted a neurology colleague who was considered the "king" of electrical activity measurement in my hospital. He thought my project was interesting and offered to let me come to his electromyography (EMG) laboratory with a patient to try out his supersensitive equipment.

I was excited. I found a patient, fifty-two years old, who was willing to offer up his poorly functioning penis for a couple of hours in the interest of science. A date was set. The day before the big test I went to the local store and sheepishly scanned the magazine racks for an, ahem, stimulating yet inoffensive source of visual sexual imagery. In other words, I bought a *Playboy* magazine. It had occurred to me that perhaps the reason I hadn't detected any electrical signal on my first try was that an erection induced with an injection might produce different electrical activity than an erection induced by being aroused. In the Danish paper, which I had reread, the authors noted that their subjects had watched an erotic videotape to stimulate an erection. A *Playboy* magazine seemed a reasonable substitute and wouldn't require any additional equipment.

The next morning I brought in the magazine hidden in a brown bag inside my briefcase. I was nervous. I was a junior faculty member. Who brings a *Playboy* to work? Worse, who shows a *Playboy* magazine to his patients? I imagined my patient being offended when I handed him the magazine to help him get aroused, and reporting me to the hospital. If not the patient, then perhaps a nurse or someone else from the EMG lab. I started to sweat. This didn't seem like such a good idea anymore.

It was still early in the morning. I called my chief, William DeWolf, MD, who had always been supportive of my work, and caught him before he started his first surgical case of the day. I told him I was planning to measure electrical activity in a man's penis.

"Interesting idea," he said encouragingly. "Why are you calling me, though?"

"Well, the man needs to get aroused to see how the electrical activity works," I explained.

"So?"

"Well, it's difficult to get aroused in a laboratory setting, so what's been done in these cases is to provide what's called 'visual sexual stimulation.'" There was silence on the other end. I just needed to say it. "I brought in a *Playboy* for the patient to look at."

"Seems reasonable to me," he said. "I've got to go. My case is about to start."

Phew! At least I had the blessing of my chief.

I met my neurology colleague, Isaac, at his lab. He proudly showed me around. The room was in an older part of the hospital, and consisted of a few connecting rooms, a waiting room, an administrative room with a secretary and walls of records. However, the heart of the operation was the EMG room itself.

In the center of the room was a standard hospital exam table. Behind it, though, was a massive rectangular piece of equipment about eight feet tall, filled with switches, gauges, knobs, and buttons. It reminded me of the very first computers I'd ever seen, as an undergraduate. "This is the most sensitive testing equipment for electric impulses in the U.S.," Isaac said with enormous pride. "There are only three allegedly equivalent devices in the entire U.S., but ours is the best. We can pick up the tiniest of electrical signals in muscles," he explained. "This room is especially designed to block out extraneous electrical activity in the building itself. If there's anything electrical happening in the penis, this baby will pick it up."

My patient Alfred arrived. I shook his hand and told him how much I appreciated his volunteering for this. He lay down on the table, dressed in the hospital gown we'd supplied, head and back slightly raised on an incline, a mildly amused expression on his face.

"Where are the electrodes?" I asked Isaac.

"Here they are," he said. They were long, thin needles, individually packed in a sterile pouch. Isaac routinely inserted these needles into muscles. Biceps, triceps, forearm, thigh, calves. Even the small muscles in the fingers. But never a penis. I had administered injections into the penis in more than one hundred men already, so that part didn't bother me much. Yet here I was, not treating anyone, just working on a project. I felt guilty but screwed up my courage. "This will only feel like a tiny prick," I said, and realized my inopportune turn of phrase as soon as I said it. So did Alfred, and we both laughed. The needle was incredibly fine, and he didn't jump at all when I inserted it.

Isaac turned on his device. There was a speaker that provided an audible signal from any detected electrical activity, but we only heard background static. There were gauges at eye level on the machine, and those read zero. And there was a continuous paper printout of the electrical activity, which now showed a flat line with occasional minor squiggles reflecting only some unavoidable background electrical "noise." "I'm pretty sure the electrical activity occurs during arousal," I explained as I handed Alfred the *Playboy* magazine. "We're going to step out of the room. I know it sounds odd, but I'd like you to try to get an erection."

Alfred started flipping through the pages of the magazine casually, as if it were nothing more interesting than *Sports Illustrated*. "This should help," he said calmly. "I guess this makes up for the needle in my dick," he joked, and we left the room. After a few minutes we knocked on the door and reentered. I lifted the sheet covering Alfred's genital region, and it sure appeared that Alfred had found something interesting to "read." However, the ticker tape still showed no activity.

Isaac turned up the gain on the device, increasing its sensitivity. "There must be many fewer muscle fibers in the penis than in the muscles we normally study," he said. "Let's see if we pick something up at this new, more sensitive setting." I checked again to make sure the needle was still in good position in Alfred's penis. We stepped out and returned a few minutes later. Still nothing. I readjusted the needle, placing it deeper within the corpora cavernosa, and we repeated the procedure. Nothing.

Isaac opened a drawer and pulled out a metal ring. "Try this," he said. "It's a different kind of sensor. Picks up surface signals, which are the cumulative signals from all the activated muscles. It is less specific, because the signal isn't from any one muscle, but it is exquisitely sensitive. We use it sometimes for small muscles, like those in the fingers."

I removed the needle from Alfred's penis and placed the new sensor around the shaft. Isaac turned the gain on the device to its most sensitive setting. We left and closed the door, again with instructions for Alfred to try to become erect. A few minutes later we heard something from the loudspeakers for the first time. Muted through the closed door, it sounded strangely like a morning traffic report on the radio. After a few minutes, we entered the room with great anticipation. As the door opened—and I will never forget this as long as I live—I heard Paul McCartney singing, "Blackbird singing in the dead of night . . ." There was no radio in the room. The music was coming from the loudspeakers on top of the big machine. I picked up the sheet covering Alfred, and saw a pretty good erection with the sensor ring still in place. Isaac was staring disbelievingly at the computer printout.

There was no mistaking it. Alfred's penis, extended by his erection and hooked up to the most supersensitive medical electrical recording device in the country, had become a radio antenna and was now channeling news, traffic, weather, and Beatles songs into this high-tech laboratory, aided and abetted by a fresh copy of *Playboy* under the auspices of my hospital and Harvard Medical School.

A year or two later I saw a follow-up article published by the same authors on electrical recordings from the penis. I didn't bother reading it. One singing penis in a lifetime was enough for me.

It's interesting to reflect back and ask how Masters and Johnson could have gotten the primary causes of ED so wrong. One lesson is that in the absence of solid information, it's difficult to come to any solid conclusions, and in the field of medicine, theories can be damaging unless based on solid conclusions. In this case, when dealing with limited information, one or two pieces of data can be overly influential.

One of the things that Masters and Johnson were proud of was that they performed in-depth interviews and physical examinations with the individuals who came to see them for treatment. When men with "impotence" were asked how they felt about sex, a great many responded in some negative way: "I don't enjoy sex anymore," or "I make sure I don't go to bed at the same time as my wife," or "When my wife tries to get something started in bed together, I tell her I have an important meeting in the morning and need my sleep." On examination these men had no obvious physical abnormalities that indicated a known cause of ED. So Masters and Johnson concluded that because there was no sign of physical impairment, and with clearcut negative attitudes about sex, these men must have a psychological basis for their problem.

What they didn't know, as did no one at the time, was how erections really worked and what made them fail. Nor could they have appreciated the fact that the vast majority of men with physical causes of ED have completely normal physical exams. The changes that occur in the corpora cavernosa with ED are far too subtle to be detected by physical examination.

Another contributing factor is that despite the increasingly permissive attitudes toward sex around that time, there was still very little information about what was "normal." Since almost no one talked about sex or their own sexual problems, a man with ED often felt as if he were a freak, the only guy on the planet with this particular problem. Masters and Johnson knew that ED wasn't particularly rare, but they had no way of knowing how common it really was. That story broke in 1994, with publication of results from the Massachusetts Male Aging Study, which studied a large population of relatively healthy men ages forty through seventy. The rate of impotence (as it was still usually called) was shocking. Overall, 52 percent of men reported some degree of impotence—mild, moderate, or total. And the numbers for men with total impotence were 5 percent at age forty and 15 percent at seventy. Masters and Johnson assumed the negative attitude about sex expressed by so many of their male patients was the *cause* of their impotence, when it actually was the *reaction* to their impotence. Of course men avoid sex if they can't get it up. It's humiliating.

7. LISTENING TO VIAGRA

Gladly I think of the days
When all my members were limber
All except one
Those days are certainly gone,
Now all my members are stiff
All except one

—JOHANN WOLFGANG VON GOETHE (1749–1832),
German poet and dramatist

Viagra was officially introduced to the world in 1998, and the impact was immediate and profound. For the first time since Man cared about his penis, that is, since the beginning of time, there was a pill that enhanced erections. Viagra obviously changed medical treatment for men with ED; however, the scope of change brought about by this little blue pill has been far broader. I have been fascinated by the way that Viagra, together with its accomplices, Cialis and Levitra, continues to shape attitudes toward male sexuality.

Unlike any prescription medicine before it, Viagra has an image, a reputation. It is the second most recognized brand name in the world, trailing only Coca-Cola. Long a staple of late-night television and stand-up comedy, Viagra is the only medication that can be a punch line to a joke and not require some explanation as to what it is. Think about it—when was the last time you heard something funny about Lipitor, the best-selling drug in the world?

The image of Viagra and the other ED pills is fairly straightforward and generally positive, the product of nearly a decade and a half of blanket marketing. The pills help a man sexually. The pills make sex fun. The pills make sex romantic. However, there is no shortage of anti-Viagra sentiment as well. The criticism can even take on a sexist, anti-male tone: "It's so typical that men would develop a Viagra for their own pleasure but leave us women without anything similar!"

But those sentiments don't capture the truth about the ED pills and their impact on men and sexuality. Spend a few hours with me in the office, and it will quickly become clear that the story is more complicated. And much more interesting.

The Promise of Sex

Alan was a fifty-three-year-old VP of sales for a large company who had seen me for several years for an elevation in the blood test PSA, which I monitored closely since this can sometimes indicate prostate cancer. Alan was a pleasant man, who never seemed to waste a minute of time. Whenever I walked into the exam room, he was always working on his laptop, reviewing presentations, or responding to e-mail. As soon as I would walk in, he would close the laptop and become immediately and fully engaged in his interaction with me.

I was curious about this latest appointment because Alan was several months early for his next scheduled visit. When I entered the room, I found him accompanied by his wife, Jeanine, whom I'd never met before. She was attractive, stylishly dressed, and appeared to be about the same age as Alan.

"What brings you to see me today?" I asked.

"Doctor, Jeanine wanted me to see you about a new problem," Alan said.

"What problem is that?"

Alan shifted in his chair. "Sex. My stuff doesn't work right anymore." Alan was clearly uncomfortable. I looked over at Jeanine. Her expression was hard to read. I noticed that the small gap between the two chairs where they sat was wider than I usually kept it. One of them had moved their chair farther away from the other.

"When you say your stuff doesn't work right anymore, what exactly do you mean?" I asked.

Alan seemed a bit flustered. "You know, I don't get hard the way I should. Sex isn't right. Jeanine isn't happy. That's why she's here with me. Hoping you can do something." In all my previous visits with Alan, he had been articulate and clear-minded, even when he was initially scared that he had prostate cancer. These short, Twitter-type messages were unusual coming from him. I again looked over at Jeanine.

"Doctor," she interjected. "Alan and I have been married for a very long time, and we've had, I would say, a very good marriage. He's worked and traveled more than I would have liked, but that's okay, he's done well, and it's made him happy. One thing I couldn't complain about is that whenever he was with me, he was really *with* me. He could leave his work behind. And when Alan came home, he was usually playful with me. If I was making dinner in the kitchen, he'd come from behind and put his arms around me, hug me, give me a kiss on the neck. And then about six months ago he started having trouble with his erections." Jeanine paused, deciding what to say next.

I looked over at Alan, who sat with elbows on his thighs, looking at the floor while Jeanine spoke.

"I enjoy sex," Jeanine continued. "We both do. And I know that Alan's high blood pressure and cholesterol issues can cause sexual problems. Of course we'd like to see if there's something you can do to help. Those ads for Viagra and Cialis are all over the television, and we're curious whether you think they might work for Alan. But the reason I insisted on coming along today is that something strange has happened with Alan. I understand he might be too embarrassed to have sex if his penis isn't responding properly. The thing that's so concerning to me, though, is that Alan has become a different person. He never touches me anymore. He never laughs. The playfulness is gone. I'm worried he's depressed, or that there's something else going on."

"Alan, what do you think?" I asked.

Alan raised his head and took a deep breath. "I'm not depressed," he said quietly. "I just don't believe a man should promise anything he can't deliver."

"What does *that* mean?" interjected Jeanine.

Alan looked at her, expressionless, and then directed his explanation to me. "If I can't have sex with Jeanine, it doesn't seem right to be physical with her. It's not fair to her."

"Alan! What are you saying?" said Jeanine, voice rising. "You don't hug me anymore because you think I'm going to cart you off to the bedroom and force you to have sex with me? Is that what you're saying? That's nuts! What do you think it's like for me to watch you go out of your way to not come near me, like I've got the plague or something? I don't care about the sex, Alan! Well, I do, but not like that. The thing I care about is us!"

Alan appeared to be physically shrinking before my eyes. He had no response for Jeanine as an awkward silence surrounded us.

When Alan and I were alone for his examination, he explained more. "I feel like I don't know how to act with Jeanine anymore. I know she'd like me to be affectionate, and I *want* to touch her. I just don't want to disappoint her more than I already have." Alan saw the hugs and kisses and everyday incidental touching between him and Jeanine as a "promise" of sex at some later time. And if he couldn't do the "ultimate deed," he felt wrong doing anything that might even hint at sex.

Alan's erections were no longer adequate for sex, and I concluded that he was a good candidate for a trial of Viagra. I wrote him a prescription.

Four weeks later Alan returned, accompanied by Jeanine. When I walked into the room, they were chatting energetically. As I took my seat they quieted and held hands. "Doctor, the Viagra works great," said Alan. "My penis works the way it's supposed to, and we're having sex again. I'm happy." He did indeed look happy.

"What makes *me* happy," said Jeanine, "is that I have my husband back. He kisses me, he hugs me. He's fun again!"

Alan's response to the ED pills was just what any doctor would want to hear. The medication not only helped him have sex but also improved his relationship with Jeanine. He's happy, she's happy—just as in the television commercials. What's clear is that within a relationship there's more to sex than just sex. In Jeanine's eyes, Alan became a much less pleasant person when he was unable to have sex. She missed the small daily instances of physical and emotional affection that are so important for keeping a relationship healthy. If it's confusing for men to know how to act like a man when everything works properly, it is almost unfathomable when a man's sexual equipment fails. Alan described it perfectly when he said he didn't know how to behave with Jeanine any longer.

The problem is compounded by men's tendency to not share their problems, especially problems that hint at any potential lack of virility. In contrast to women, who have created community, education, and even comedy around their biology of aging (witness the off-Broadway play *Menopause The Musical*), men rarely have the opportunity to discuss how to cope with "personal" problems, like ED. Men may share with other guys that they've taken Viagra or Cialis, but it is always with the implicit understanding that they did it to enhance the experience and not because they had an actual problem that required medical treatment. The one exception is men who have survived cancer treatments. In those cases men are often quite outspoken about what they've needed to do to be sexual. "Fighting cancer" is a manly enough endeavor so that some can admit to the side effects of treatment, without impotence necessarily reflecting on their manhood.

In the absence of good modeling, men with ED sometimes behave strangely, in ways that can appear hurtful to their partners and difficult for women to understand. Alan's withdrawal of physical touching and other forms of affection is not unusual. For some men any kind of physical contact reminds them of their perceived inadequacy. In Alan's case, he shut down all touching, kissing, and other forms of physical affection because he thought it was *the only fair thing to do* for Jeanine. Overpromising is a major violation of trust and is a recipe for an unhappy relationship. The problem here, of course, is that a relationship with one's spouse is not the same as with a business client. Even more important, touching, kissing, and hugging may sometimes lead to sex, but they don't have to, and they can be pleasurable in their own way.

It's difficult for many men to verbalize their feelings of inadequacy and their fears, yet if Alan had been able to do so, Jeanine could have reassured him that she still wanted to be close to him physically. The coldness and hostility between the two of them would never have developed, and Alan could still have sought help for his ED without Jeanine feeling that Alan found her repulsive, or that he'd undergone a change in his personality.

Breast Is Okay, *Nipple* Is Not

There have been any number of new, potential blockbuster medications rolled out by big pharmaceutical companies over the last quarter century, but I don't recall anything quite the same as Viagra. Attention by the public, the media, and even by the business community was over the top. Everyone was interested. A miracle pill for sex? What a story!

I remember being interviewed about this new wonder pill for a local TV station. It was always challenging to speak delicately about guy "stuff" while still trying to be clear. Talking about Viagra and what it did was going to be particularly tough if I had to dance around the issue. So as we prepared for the interview, I had a pow-wow with my interviewer. "Can I use the words *penis* and *erection*?" I asked.

The female correspondent was experienced and well respected. She thought about it for a quick second. "You have to," she said. "I don't see how you can say anything useful about Viagra without using those words. Everyone knows by now what Viagra does anyway." Then she added, "There is an interesting parallel in women's health. Only a few years ago we couldn't use the word *breast* on television because it was considered too sexual. However, with the rise in breast cancer awareness and recommendations from so many doctors for mammograms, the walls had to come down. So now we say *breast* all the time."

"I never realized that," I said.

"Yes. But we still never use the word *nipple!*" she added with a chuckle. "*Nipple* is still considered too sexual!"

How far we've come. The other evening I was flipping channels on television and came across a rerun of the popular comedy *Two and Half Men*. I had never seen the show and decided to watch for a few minutes. The setup for the show is that two brothers, Charlie and Alan Harper, live together, Alan is divorced, and his son lives with them part-time. The scene I saw amazed me. Alan (played by the actor Jon Cryer) walks into the living room late at night, where Charlie (played by Charlie Sheen) is watching television. When Alan complains that he can't sleep, Charlie says to him flatly, "Why don't you go back to your room and just masturbate?"

Alan: "I already tried that. Didn't work." (Canned laughter)

Charlie: "Thanks for telling me. I'm glad I didn't shake your hand when you came out." (Canned laughter)

There's very little I haven't heard, but I confess I was shocked. This was national television programming during family hour!

It's difficult for me to accept the idea that this crude attempt at humor represents any kind of social advance. Nonetheless, it is undeniable that our culture has become radically more accepting of sexual talk. I firmly believe that the introduction of Viagra contributed enormously to this change, for good or ill.

From the moment Viagra alighted on the social consciousness there was a new conversation at every imaginable forum about men, sex, and erections—around water coolers, in bedrooms, on commuter trains. Only a few months earlier, the rallying cry for physicians like me was to encourage men to talk about their sexual problems. "It's okay," we would say, "the problem is common and usually physical. It's nothing to be ashamed of." With Viagra men by the thousands came out of the darkness, curious, relieved, sometimes desperate.

The marketing folks did an impressive job with Viagra from the get-go. They knew there was a huge number of men who could benefit from it, but they needed to overcome a culture of shame for men with impotence. They took a brilliant step, hiring Bob Dole to be their first spokesperson. Senator Dole was the Republican candidate for president in 1996, and it was public knowledge that he'd undergone a radical prostatectomy for prostate cancer, an operation which causes erection problems in many men. Imagine—here was a man who could have been president of the United States just two years earlier, talking about Viagra. By having Bob Dole talk about it and give the impression he used it, there was no longer any reason why "regular" folks couldn't do the same.

Shortly after the FDA's approval of Viagra, a sixtyish orthopedic surgeon approached me in the lounge where surgeons and operating room staff congregated between cases for coffee or lunch. I knew him by name, but we'd never spoken.

"I wonder if you could help me," he said. "I have a patient who I think would do well with Viagra. Can you tell me how to write the prescription?"

I chuckled quietly to myself. Orthopedists are notorious for treating nothing outside their surgical specialty. Only in street language could ED be seen as a "bone problem." This was just like a high school student asking the teacher for help for "a friend" in trouble, who in reality is the student himself. It was obvious to me that the surgeon wanted the Viagra for himself. I instructed him on dosage and other details, and wished him luck with his patient. He thanked me and then stepped away. Over the years I ran into him many times in the same surgery lounge. He would nod his head hello but never chatted with me again.

The Sex Appeal of Baseball

Nathan, a forty-eight-year-old man, saw me for ED. He was married and hadn't been able to have sex in two years. Erections were poor with masturbation too, and he never awakened with a firm erection any more. I prescribed Viagra for him and gave him the usual set of instructions. Give it thirty to sixty minutes to get into your system before sex, take it on an empty stomach (absorption is slowed considerably by food or alcohol), and make sure to do something sexual. Nathan thanked me and made an appointment to see me in a month, giving him time to really try the medication.

At Nathan's follow-up visit, he shook his head, pursed his lips, and said to me, "Doc, that stuff doesn't work."

"What do you mean?" I asked.

"I tried it and nothing happened."

"Tell me exactly how you took it."

"Doc, I did just what you told me. I took it in the evening, *before* dinner, just like you said, so my stomach would be empty. Then I went to the living room to watch the baseball game to give it time to work, just like you told me. My wife was in the bedroom, waiting for me in case something happened. I watched the whole baseball game, and nothing happened."

"Did you try to have sex?"

"No. Like I told you, I never got a hard-on, so there wasn't any point in trying."

Well, Nathan hadn't *quite* followed my instructions. In contrast to penile injections, in which the penis becomes pharmacologically "activated," the ED pills do not cause erections on their own. Men need to be sexually aroused or stimulated to see any effect from the ED pills. Nathan was never going to get a Viagra-enhanced erection by watching the Boston Red Sox on television unless he happened to be strangely excited by double plays and home runs.

This feature of the pills is fortuitous. Otherwise, any man who, in anticipation of "getting lucky," took one of the ED pills before going out in public would be saddled with a premature, embarrassing erection, drawing attention to himself wherever he went.

The way the ED pills work is really quite remarkable. During most of the day, when the penis is flaccid, there is barely a trickle of blood flow into the penis. However, with arousal or sexual stimulation the smooth muscle lining the arteries and the tissues of the penis relax, and blood flow to the penis is greatly increased. Viagra and the other pills have nothing to do with this initial erectile response. What they do is interfere with the breakdown of the signal that leads to erection, which results in a stronger signal. That chemical signal is called cyclic guanosine monophosphate, or cGMP, and cGMP is broken down to an inactive form by an enzyme called phosphodiesterase (PDE). Phosphodiesterases are found throughout the body, but by luck, at least for men and the makers of the ED pills, there is a specific form of PDE that is found almost exclusively within the corpora cavernosa, called type 5. What Viagra and the other pills do is inhibit the activity of this enzyme, which is why this class of medication is called PDE5 inhibitors.

Practically speaking, what all this biochemical mumbo-jumbo means is that the pills aren't involved in *creating* the signal for erection; the man has to generate that on his own with sexual thoughts or actions. Once the man creates his own chemical signal within the penis, the pills take over from there.

The Exuberant Administrator

Carl was a married, sixty-four-year-old administrator who had come to see me for erectile dysfunction, accompanied by his wife, Elysse, an attractive, well-dressed woman of sixty-two. "This coming July we'll have been married forty years," Carl announced proudly. Carl had noticed his erections waning for several years. He was relatively healthy but carried an extra fifty pounds, which seemed to have settled primarily in his midsection. He was on medication for elevated cholesterol and triglycerides.

When I asked Carl how I could help him, it was Elysse who answered: "Doctor, we have a very good marriage." She looked toward Carl to indicate they were speaking as one. "And we've always been very affectionate with each other. I've always been very open about the physical part of our relationship, and I understood when things stopped working for Carl the way they used to. These things happen. We've done our reading, and we understand this is almost certainly a physical issue for Carl. So we'd like to know what you can do to help Carl. Physically, that is. If you can help, great. If not, then I guess this is where we are in life." Elysse spoke calmly, as if she'd worked this all through in her mind.

"Carl, anything you'd like to add?" I asked.

"Elysse summed it up pretty well," he said. "I guess I'd be interested in trying one of the pills that are advertised on TV all the time."

For most men with ED, the PDE5 inhibitors are a very reasonable first choice. They have proven to be very safe, although many men do experience nuisance-type side effects, such as headache, nasal congestion, heartburn, and facial flushing. The most important safety issue is that men who take nitrate medications for heart disease should not take PDE5 inhibitors, as the combination with nitrates can trigger a dangerous drop in blood pressure.

Once I had examined Carl and reviewed his test results, which confirmed a physical ED, I handed him a prescription for Viagra and gave him the usual instructions, then added, "And remember to try to do something sexual—if you don't, you're unlikely to see any effect."

"Thanks, Doctor," Carl replied. He seemed eager to try the pills and get started.

A month or so later Carl returned to the office, alone, to report on how well the medication had worked. "The pills work," he said, despondently.

"That should be good news," I said, puzzled, "but you don't seem very happy about it. Is everything all right?"

"Elysse doesn't want me to take the pills anymore," Carl replied. "She says sex is supposed to be a natural and spontaneous event between two people who care for each other. She'd rather have no sex at all than have us plan ahead." Carl sighed. "I probably brought this on myself. I talked too much with her about how I was supposed to take it, empty stomach and all that. I'm frustrated because the pills were good. I took the Viagra twice, and it was the first two times we've had real sex in over a year. I was proud of myself," he said, looking up at me with the saddest smile imaginable.

"Elysse didn't say anything the first time. Maybe she didn't want to burst my bubble. After the second time, a few days later, she told me she wasn't comfortable with it. She can get pretty stubborn too, once she gets an idea in her mind. I wish I could do it naturally, like she wants, but I can't. Now I'm stuck. I don't know what to do. I wonder if I'll ever have sex again."

Elysse's complaints about the ED pills are common. Taking a pill ahead of time does spoil the idea of romantic, unscheduled, spontaneous sex. For nearly all men with ED, though, it's an easy choice between planned sex with the pills versus no sex at all! I had a possible solution for Carl that might be acceptable to Elysse.

A few years ago Cialis came up with a novel approach to the problem, which was to take a small dose of Cialis every single day. Cialis stays in the body longer than Viagra and Levitra, and the scientists at Lilly, which makes Cialis, figured out that by taking a small dose every day, men could maintain a fairly constant and effective concentration of Cialis in their bloodstream that would help them have sex just as if they had taken a larger pill the usual way. The beauty of this approach was that no planning for sex was necessary. The man was ready to go, anytime at all. Daily low-dose Cialis comes close to being a real cure for ED for many men, although they must obviously continue to take the medication daily.

Carl was eager to try daily Cialis. I saw him back in the office a month later. When I walked into the room, he stood up and actually hugged me. He was so ecstatic that I thought he was going to do cartwheels in the hallway. "Cialis did the trick! Elysse still isn't crazy about me taking a medicine for sex, but we don't have to plan anything anymore. She even seems to like me again! I'm so relieved. Oh my god, I never thought I'd say something like this, with all the negative press about how the drug companies are tainting medicine, but . . . long live pharmaceuticals!"

I was happy for Carl and couldn't suppress a grin while he was telling me what had happened. Just goes to show what restoring a man's sex life will do for him!

Round Three

Cecil was a forty-two-year-old entrepreneur who made an appointment to see me for "erection problems," as he wrote on his medical intake form. "I'm here to see if I can get some of that Cialis," he said when we met.

"Are you having trouble with erections?" I asked.

"Yes and no," he answered.

"What do you mean?"

"Well, I'm single, and I do a lot of dating," he began. "I like women who are a lot younger than me, women in their midtwenties, usually." Cecil stopped, as if what he'd said was enough of an explanation, but my blank expression told him I needed more information.

"You see, the younger women these days, at least the women I date, they're very demanding sexually. My erection is fine for round one, and usually for round two, but I can't get it going for round three anymore."

"If I understand you correctly," I said, "your erection is perfectly fine the first time you have sex and even the second time in an evening. Is that right?"

"Right," he said, head nodding, happy that I now seemed to be following him.

"And the reason you're here is that you want to be able to go for three rounds instead of two?"

"*Right,*" he said, drawing out the word, as if I weren't so dense after all.

"Cecil, most guys in their forties would be thrilled to have sex twice in one evening. What makes you feel that twice isn't enough?"

"That just doesn't seem right, Doc. I'm in great shape. The women all think I'm in my early thirties. I don't see why I can't have sex three times like I used to."

"Cecil, it's normal for men to take longer to recharge as they age," I explained. "I'm not saying you're old, not by any means, but men at forty-two like you aren't the same as when they were twenty-two. It takes longer to get the next erection and sometimes even longer than that to be able to come again. I have plenty of patients your age who are also in great shape who only have sex once a night, and then they're done. They couldn't have another erection if the most beautiful woman in the world walked into their bedroom. And there's nothing wrong with them."

"That's sick, man," Cecil said, shaking his head.

"It's just what happens. That time to recharge the battery is called the refractory period, and one of the things about men and sex is that the refractory period gets longer as they get older. Some teenage boys can come seven or eight times a day, no problem, but that's not true as they get older."

"Doc, listen. In the crowd I run with, these women expect a

lot. If I can't get with them more than twice, they'll just kick me to the curb."

"Cecil, I find it hard to believe that if a woman were really interested in you, she would drop you because you can only have sex twice in a night."

"Doc," Cecil explained as if I were a poor soul who just did not get it, "this isn't about love. This is about sex. Just sex, pure and simple."

We talked some more, but I wasn't comfortable writing Cecil a prescription. He didn't have ED, and I was unsympathetic to his circumstances. Perhaps I would have felt differently if he'd told me that he was really crazy about this one woman and he felt he needed it until their relationship could blossom in other ways. It seemed to me that Cecil was trying to prove he was still a young stud, to himself or to these nameless women, and that didn't seem like an adequate reason to prescribe the medication.

"I'm sorry, Cecil, I can't give you that prescription. Medically, you're okay. In fact, you're doing better than most men your age."

"That's okay, Doc," he said. "I understand. I figured I'd try with you. I'll get Cialis from another doctor. Or maybe from the Internet," and off he went.

Shy Penis

Alexander was a twenty-seven-year-old graduate student who wrote on his medical intake form that the reason he was here to see me was that he had a "shy penis." When we sat down together, he explained. "I always have trouble when I start seeing a girl. I can feel my penis get hard when we make out, but the first couple of times I try to actually have sex with a girl, my penis is always soft. If the girl likes me enough to stick around, eventually it starts working, and I've always been totally fine when I've had a steady girlfriend. It's been this way since I first started having sex, or at least trying to have sex, when I was twenty. It's embarrassing, though. And there have been a couple of girls that just thought it was too weird that I couldn't do it with them, so they didn't stick around. There was one in particular, about two years ago, that I still think of. I thought we had a really good connection."

Alexander had clear-cut, classic psychogenic ED. He and I both understood that there was nothing physically wrong with him. Yet he was hoping that by using Viagra he could have successful sex right away, when the moment presented itself, instead of floundering around for a while.

This use of Viagra, and later, the other pills, for young healthy men with psychogenic ED was a serious "bone" of contention early on. I remember lecturing to a group of approximately one hundred physicians in Copenhagen soon after Viagra's introduction. I did an informal poll of who among them would treat with Viagra in hypothetical situations by asking for a show of hands. The first case was a sixty-year-old smoker with hypertension, high cholesterol, and diabetes (all of which are risk factors for ED) who was married and had been experiencing progressive difficulties achieving an adequate erection over three years. Everyone raised their hand.

Next I asked about a twenty-five-year-old man whose story was similar to Alexander's. His erections were fine, but he became anxious before having sex the first time with a new partner. It was a clear case of psychogenic ED. Who would treat this man? Not one of the doctors raised their hand. Then I asked how many would treat him if he returned to the office after having failed three times with the same woman. Only one or two hands went up. I asked the audience why they were so reluctant to treat in this case. A middle-aged doctor in the first row stood up. "The young man's problem is clearly psychological," he said. "He doesn't need a pill. He needs to learn to relax, just like we all did at that age." There was a cheerful murmuring of agreement. "This young man needs to take a drink, get to know the girl better, and get counseling if nothing else helps. There is nothing wrong with him, and I would not give him a prescription medicine for this problem."

Many physicians stateside had a similar response when Viagra first appeared, reserving the medication only for those cases where there was a clear-cut physical cause. I never agreed with that approach. These days, many couples have sex very early in a relationship. It takes a long time to really get to know someone, but it is not unusual for sex to take place on a first, second, or third date. It is as if couples now begin their relationships with sex and then figure out whether they even like each other.

Moreover, we have this romantic, idealized notion that sexual attractiveness and compatibility are critical components of a desirable relationship. If sex doesn't work out, maybe it just wasn't meant to be. When sex doesn't work out between two individuals who don't know each other very well, there is a strong possibility that the twosome won't become a couple. If the erection fails, a woman may worry that she doesn't turn him on or, more selfishly, may think to herself, "I can't be with a man who can't have sex with me." For the man, his sexual failure is usually experienced as shame, and consciously or unconsciously he many not want to put himself in that situation again. He may well have performed fine with a prior girlfriend, and he thinks, "Heck, we just don't click." All of this puts a lot of pressure on a man to have his penis work properly at the beginning of a relationship.

Despite this pressure, I have seen so many cases where there was a "false start" to the sexual part of the relationship initially, but it went on be a loving and very good sexual relationship. One of the reasons I've been open to the idea of treating men with psychogenic ED of this type is that I believe the treatment, if successful, may become the key to the most significant event of a man's life. I don't mean that the man will have the best sex of his life. Rather, that successful sex may lead to a great, new relationship. For most men and women, our primary intimate relationships have the greatest impact on our lives. Especially for younger individuals, those relationships become our new family units and determine whether we go through life feeling loved, valued, supported. We often define ourselves and evaluate our lives in later years in terms of those relationships: "I was a good husband or wife" or "I was a good father or mother."

Sex is not just sex, then. It is a necessary component to the beginning of many relationships, and I believe that by providing a treatment for the "shy penis," I am potentially helping a man find love and happiness. The cause of the difficulty in these men is simple: anxiety. We've come so far from the attitudes of Masters and Johnson and the zeitgeist of several decades ago. One doesn't have to invoke a complex mother-child relationship when a man fails to have an adequate erection with a new partner. It's just scary. And it's not difficult to understand why.

Sex is weird. It is unlike anything else we do. We break rule after traditional rule when we have sex. In mainstream U.S. culture there is almost no physical touching or affection between individuals who aren't sexual partners. It shouldn't be surprising that men may have trouble getting an erection with a new partner. Indeed, it is surprising that sex ever works out in the first place!

Since Viagra first arrived on the scene, I've prescribed it for many men with anxiety-related ED. My instructions to them are different than to men with physical causes of ED. The goal is to create a belief that sex will work out fine, to create positive expectations to replace the negative ones: "Sex is great!" instead of "Oh no, she's going to be so pissed if I fail again." I tell the men to use the medication at full dose and to use it every single time they try to have sex for the next three months. What invariably happens is that the men abandon the pills soon after. Once they start having successful intercourse, there will be an occasion where sex happens spontaneously, before they've had time to take the pill, and at that point they realize they don't need it anymore. I believe many potentially good relationships will not survive a prolonged period of sexual difficulties at the beginning; why not give a man the chance to see if the woman he's dating might be his perfect partner?

Most people assume that the ED pills always work, and that a man can be sexual into his nineties. The very first large study to be published, in the *New England Journal of Medicine*, reported a success rate of approximately 80 percent. This high success rate became part of the lore about Viagra. Not emphasized was that the men who received a placebo had a success rate of almost 50 percent. Pfizer had selected a highly favorable group of men for their first study, men who were likely to respond to Viagra. Men with purely physical ED were excluded from the study. This was why so many in the placebo group did well.

However, as physicians gained experience and performed additional studies in men with exclusively physical causes of ED, the success rate dropped considerably. Today, most studies show a similar success rate for all three of the pills of about 65 percent, with lower success rates of approximately 50 percent in some groups, such as diabetics and in men following prostate cancer treatment. That's still a very good success rate, but it's far from a guarantee.

I've always had a fondness for clever advertising, and I've already mentioned the Bob Dole campaign for Viagra. One of the later Viagra ads on TV was also a favorite of mine. A man walks through his office, quietly confident and cheerful, while his workmates watch him and ask, "What's different about Bob?"

"Is it his glasses?"

"Is it his hair?"

"Is it his clothes?"

As Bob exits the office he looks back with a knowing smile, and the word *Viagra* appears onscreen in large letters. There *is* something different about men who have regained their sexuality, even if we have trouble putting our finger on what that quality may be.

The most recent campaign provides a different message. In one television commercial, we see a middle-aged, nice-looking man sailing alone contentedly. A rope snaps, and the sail flutters awkwardly. Unperturbed, the sailor improvises by finding a strap in the hold and rerigs the sail. He pulls in to dock as the sun sets, and drives his truck to a pleasant, modest home with the lights on. A wry smile comes across his face, and he heads to the front door as the word *Viagra* comes onscreen. The message is clear: men deal with problems. Erectile dysfunction is just another problem, and Viagra is the solution. A Viagra print ad tells the same message: "This is the age of knowing who you are. You've been there, lived that, and learned from it. So, why would you let something like erectile dysfunction (ED) get in your way? If you're like millions of men who have some degree of ED, talk to your doctor about Viagra."

It is a modern message, one that I echo in this book. ED eventually affects nearly all men. It doesn't make one less of a man, and there are effective treatments. So, as the Viagra ads suggest, "deal with it."

For me, the Viagra era has provided a window into the psyche of men. The stories men share speak powerfully of the importance of sex to a man's sense of his own manhood and reveal just as much about how men view their sexuality within relationships.

Men care deeply about how they are regarded by their partners, sexually and otherwise. Alan's soft penis, for example, did not prevent him from enjoying the pleasure and comfort of Jeanine's kisses and hugs, or even from having an orgasm. He wanted to behave in an honorable way with Jeanine, which in his own convoluted way of thinking meant that he needed to cut off all affection and physical contact. Viagra restored Alan's erections and his ability to have sex, which in turn made Alan feel as if he again had permission to be affectionate with Jeanine. This restoration of his manhood via his erection also subtly changed his behavior in other ways: he was happy again, playful, generous, teasing. Men who are comfortable with their manliness have access to a wide range of positive feelings and behaviors. Perhaps this is what John Lennon meant in the Beatles song lyric "Happiness is a warm gun."

Simple things are no longer so simple for men. Is it all right to open a door for a woman, or is that sexist? Pay for dinner when your date has a better job? How does a man pull off the magical feat of appearing strong yet sensitive at the same time? Yet these and other questions of our time pale in comparison to questions about the secret world of sex. Is it okay to make the first move? To be forceful or demanding? Is it demeaning to talk dirty to one's partner? Once we add in erection problems, men may be at a complete loss about how to act, and it is no wonder that some of the choices they make create new difficulties within relationships.

When we consider the incredible impact that losing and then regaining erections has on men, when we really listen to Viagra, we learn something rather remarkable. For the man within a relationship, even if he is incapable of saying a single affectionate word, sex is the way that he communicates his commitment and, yes, love.

8. A HUSBAND'S DUTY

We only know of one duty, and that is to love.
—ALBERT CAMUS (1913–60), French writer

Once something new comes along, it is difficult to imagine life without it. On my bookshelf sits a massive copy of the unabridged Random House dictionary, a gift I bought myself from my first paycheck. Today it stands, untouched in years, replaced by the Internet. My college-age daughters cannot imagine how much planning was necessary to meet friends before everyone had a cell phone. Arrangements required precise timing and specific, easily recognized landmarks, or else the rendezvous would never take place. Today, it is enough for my daughters to text their friends "See you around 3p at the mall," without concerns for missing each other due to near-constant status updates ("Leaving house now. U?").

In the world of sexuality Viagra is the genie we cannot put back in the bottle. With recognition that most ED is physical, not psychological, the emotional burden was relieved. However, by itself this did nothing to solve the underlying problem; men with ED still had ED. A variety of new treatments were being developed and explored, yet none were especially easy or appealing to use. Indeed, the challenge of finding a successful and acceptable treatment for men with ED during this period contributed greatly to my view of men and sexuality. It's when the stakes are highest that we learn what people are really all about.

A Guy Thing

It was the early 1990s when Jose came to see me, accompanied by his wife, Rita. Jose was a forty-seven-year-old building custodian; Rita, forty-five, cared for their three children and also worked part-time pressing clothes at a dry-cleaning outlet. The couple resembled each other with round faces, round bodies—both were considerably overweight—and big smiles. "Doctor, I don't have any trouble *getting* hard," explained Jose. "My problem is I can't *stay* hard. My penis gets soft after a couple of minutes, sometimes before I even have a chance to put it in. I know what's happening in bed is frustrating for her, and she deserves better. I hope you can do something to help me. To help *us*."

When it was still uncommon to identify a physical source for ED, one of the few physical excuses for it was severe arterial disease from atherosclerosis. Clogged arteries. In those cases, the standard story was that men couldn't *get* hard. The problem of *staying* hard, as Jose described, was considered indicative of psychogenic impotence.

Take, for example, the man who maintains a firm erection while making out on the couch, fully clothed, but loses his erection as soon as he slips naked under the sheets in anticipation of actual sex. Or a man who loses his erection as soon as he attempts to put on a condom. In these cases the man loses his erection due to anticipation of what is about to happen, and today we would just call this performance anxiety.

Jose's assessment of his own problem was insightful. "Doctor, Rita read in a magazine that this problem is usually psychological." Jose glanced at Rita, and smiled. "But I don't think there's anything wrong with my mind. Well"—he chuckled—"maybe there is, but it doesn't affect *this*. To me, it feels like there's something wrong with my penis, like it won't hold the blood inside. It feels like a tire with an air leak." He smiled again as he made this surprisingly accurate analogy.

Jose was right on the mark. Once we had injections to create involuntary, pharmacological erections, we were able to study not only how erections worked but also how they failed. And one of the surprising things we learned was that the most common problem was not choked arterial supply to the penis but an inadequate trapping of blood *within* the penis, which was a problem of the veins. The penis has a special mechanism to compress the veins during erection, allowing the penis to maintain rigidity with only minimal additional inflow from the arteries. When the internal venous compression mechanism doesn't work well, too much blood exits through the veins, causing the penis to soften. The technical term is veno-occlusive dysfunction, but it is more frequently referred to as a venous leak. Jose's analogy of a tire with an air leak was entirely apt. Today we know, from studies performed during that era, that approximately 80 percent of men with a physical cause of ED have a venous leak as the root cause.

Jose's symptoms were classic for this problem. The early excitement phase of normal erections brings a rapid increase of blood into the corpora cavernosa via the arteries. The blood fills the corpora cavernosa, the penis expands, and veins lying just underneath the tunica albuginea become compressed by the expanded penile tissue pressing against the tough tunica albuginea. This compression causes the veins to collapse, reducing their ability to allow blood to escape the corpora cavernosa. In men with venous leak, the penile tissues have lost some of their elasticity, preventing the veins from being adequately compressed, and blood escapes. If the leak is small, the penis may remain reasonably firm but as the leak becomes larger, the penis may fill initially with the rush of new blood, but then soften over time, and when the leak is very large, the penis may never become firm at all.

I had some more questions for Jose. "Jose, how is your desire for sex these days?" I asked.

"Strong!" he responded, smiling.

"How often do the two of you do something sexual together?"

"Three, maybe four times a week," he answered. Rita nodded her head in agreement.

This was good news. Many men who experience problems with erections usually start to shy away from sex due to frustration or embarrassment. The fact that Jose and Rita kept up this level of frequent sexual activity at this point in their marriage and with Jose's difficulties indicated that sex was something they both enjoyed together.

"Jose, I'm curious about something. Since you and Rita still play around sexually a few times a week, why do you feel you still need treatment?"

Rita looked over at Jose, waiting with great interest to hear how he would respond.

Jose looked at me as if he couldn't believe I could ask a question with such an obvious answer. "Doctor," he began, "it's not right to be this way. I feel terrible that I can't be more of a man for my wife."

"Rita, what do you think about what Jose just said?" I asked.

Rita was quick to respond. "I don't know what he's talking about. Of course I'd like it if we could have sex again like we used to, but Jose doesn't need to do anything special to prove to me he's a man. He's a great father and a great husband." She turned to face Jose and spoke to him in a gentle, quieter tone, as if I weren't there. "What are you saying, baby? You know how I feel. You don't have to do any of this for me." Their eyes met, and Jose turned away, eyes moist.

"I'm just telling the doctor how I feel, that's all," he said quietly. Rita put her arm through Jose's and leaned into him.

As you may have noticed, Jose's description of how he felt was typical of the responses I've heard from so many men in similar circumstances. This feeling about one's masculinity has nothing to do with sexual conquests, the frequency of sex, or unusual sexual positions. It is about service to the woman. Doing right by one's partner. In my experience, nearly all men believe that "doing right" by the woman sexually requires a hard penis and the ability to have intercourse the old-fashioned way, that is, penis inside vagina.

Rita's response to Jose was what we all dream about hearing from our partners—that they acknowledge and love us, as we are and as we may have changed with time, regardless of what we may regard as our own shortcomings or failures. The feeling that Jose's erection problem negatively reflected his masculinity came from inside Jose's own head, from his own internal belief system about what men are supposed to do, and how they are supposed to be.

Men express the same sentiment even when the woman is perfectly satisfied with their sexual relationship. Many women are able to have an orgasm only with manual or oral stimulation, others may experience pain with insertion of the penis into the vagina, and others may not even enjoy sex at all. Yet their male partners remain convinced of the importance of the firm penis for vaginal insertion.

In the pre–birth control era when it was widely assumed that women were not intended to enjoy sex, there was a curious term, *performing one's wifely duty*, which referred to the assumed obligation of married women to submit graciously to their husband's unpleasant and insistent requests for sex. Since the women's movement, they have enjoyed the power of having sex only when they want to, and the *wifely duty* term has been relegated to the wastebasket of history. I believe that listening to men and their attitudes about sexuality and masculinity has made this a propitious time to coin an analogous term for men: a *husband's duty* to provide sexually for his partner. Though not as unpleasant as a *wifely duty*, it does reflect the feeling men have about their responsibility to satisfy their wives.

This is no small thing. Today, a man who feels bad about how he fulfills his *husbandly duty* due to ED can request a prescription for Viagra or Cialis from his physician, or even obtain some, anonymously, via the Internet. Before Viagra, though, the stakes were much higher, since treatment was more invasive and unpleasant. Nonetheless, men like Jose still sought to meet their need to feel good about themselves as sexual providers to their wives or girlfriends, demonstrating the powerful masculine imperative to be a sexual provider as part of the successful male experience.

A brief note about the ED pills marketed via the Internet. Several studies have shown that nearly all of these are counterfeit products, most produced in Third World countries, providing only a fraction of the labeled dose of the active ingredients. Even more concerning, chemical analysis revealed that several of these were found to contain dangerous contaminants. In one study, none of the pills alleged to come from "Canadian pharmacies" were actually shipped from Canada. Caveat emptor.

After obtaining some tests I met with Jose to discuss the results. "Jose," I said, "the results of your tests show that your erection problem is due to poor trapping of blood in the penis. It's physical, and it's very much like what you described when I first met you, like air escaping from a tire. We call this a venous leak of the penis."

Jose seemed proud he had made his own diagnosis. "What can I do about it?" he asked.

"There are a few choices," I explained. "The most common treatment for men with erection problems is to learn how to inject medicine into your penis. It's very effective. Most men get a really firm erection that can last for a long time—thirty minutes, an hour, sometimes longer."

Jose stopped me and leaned forward in his seat. "You're kidding. Does it hurt?"

"No. The needle is so small you would barely feel it."

Jose was trying to wrap his brain about this new concept. "Does that mean I would need to come here to get an injection every time I wanted to have sex?" he asked incredulously.

"No." I chuckled. "We would teach you how to do it yourself. I can't be available every Friday or Saturday night when you want to get busy!" I joked.

Jose sat back again. He didn't seem particularly interested in injections. "What else can I do?"

"There is something called a vacuum device. It's a plastic cylinder that goes over the penis, and a pump sucks out the air. Blood runs into the penis, and it gets pretty hard. Then a band goes onto the base of the penis to keep the blood inside and the penis hard. You have sex with the band at the base of your penis."

Jose was shaking his head throughout my description. This wasn't for him. "Anything else?" he asked.

"There's an operation I can do to place a device within the penis, called an implant, or penile prosthesis. Two hollow cylinders go inside your own two natural cylinders where erection normally takes place. When you want to have sex, you squeeze a little pump within the scrotum—it's like a third testicle—and water fills the cylinders, making the penis stand up. It's just like a normal erection, except the cylinders are filled with water instead of blood. The penis stands up and gets just as firm, sometimes firmer, as a natural erection. When you're finished, you squeeze a different spot, and the penis goes back down again."

"Doctor, I'm not afraid of surgery, but isn't there anything you can do so I can have my own erections without all these gadgets?"

"Maybe. There is a fairly new procedure in which the leaking veins are tied off. If it works, you will get your own good erections at the beginning, as you do already, and the penis will then stay firm for a longer time."

"That's what I'm looking for," said Jose. "Do whatever you need to do. This is important to me."

It was an exciting time in the world of sexual medicine. Brindley and Virag not only had provided a new form of treatment for ED with penile injections but had also provided a means to evaluate the penis under laboratory conditions. The second procedure I had mentioned to Jose was called penile venous ligation. (*Liga-*

tion means tying something off.) The procedure had been developed only a few years before, and the results were uneven. New data indicated that better rates of success could be expected with specific patterns of venous drainage from the penis, and I needed to find out whether Jose was in a favorable category. If not, I would be reluctant to put him through the operation.

It's incredible to me now to reflect on what we did back then to evaluate men with ED. My small fraternity of colleagues in sexual medicine from around the United States and beyond were determined to do what we could to base the exciting new treatments on actual numbers and facts. Erections were a vascular event mediated by blood vessels, and one should therefore be able to apply laboratory techniques to the penis that were borrowed from cardiac and other vascular assessments. The study of blood flow in the heart and major blood vessels by cardiologists is called hemodynamics; my field now had *penodynamics*.

Jose arrived in a special procedure room set up for interventional radiologists, where a variety of procedures were performed that required fluoroscopy, a type of real-time X-ray. He lay down on the table. A blood pressure monitor was attached to his arm, and EKG leads to his chest. A sterile drape was then placed over Jose's body, with a small opening through which I would have access to his penis.

I put on a sterile gown and gloves, and then injected the penis with local anesthesia just behind the corona (crown), the ridge behind the head of penis (the glans). Once the penis was numb I placed monitoring needles into each of the corpora cavernosa. I then injected vasodilators into the penis to "activate" it, creating an erection, just as Brindley had done to himself.

With sophisticated equipment, I determined the pressure within the penile arteries and the speed with which blood left the corpora cavernosa via the veins. Jose had a clear-cut venous leak of moderate severity. His arteries were fine.

Next came the X-ray part of the test to determine the pattern

of venous drainage from the corpora cavernosa. I injected contrast material into the corpora cavernosa via one of the needles
I'd placed at the beginning of the study. This contrast material
looks white on X-rays, as bones do, and can therefore light up the
veins draining the penis if the contrast material gets into them. In
men with good venous trapping, all the contrast stays within the
corpora cavernosa themselves and none is seen in the veins leaving the penis. When a venous leak is present, the contrast within
the veins makes them show up on X-rays like white worms. The
latest research indicated that the venous ligation operation worked
best in men whose leak arose from the outermost portion of the
penis. If it leaked from deeper, in the portion of the penis that
extended underneath the scrotum, the procedure almost never
worked.

I injected contrast into Jose's penis and took X-rays from various angles. Sure enough, contrast was seen lighting up several
of the veins leading away from the penis, visually confirming the
presence of a venous leak. Those veins were all from the outer
part of the penis. Jose was a good candidate for the surgery.

I gave Jose the news as I removed the needles from his penis
and applied a mild compression bandage.

"That's great, Doctor!" exclaimed Jose as he sat up on the side
of the procedure table. "How soon can you do the operation?"

"Jose, there are a few things I need to tell you about this procedure before we schedule it. First, it's pretty new, and if it works for
you, I don't know how long the benefits may last. Second, I have
to tell you that I've only performed a dozen or so cases so far."

"How did those men do?" Jose asked.

"So far, so good," I answered. "Three-quarters of the men are
pleased that their erections are firmer and last longer. The rest
didn't have any benefit at all."

"What about risks?"

"The biggest risk is you might go through the procedure and
not see any improvement. In fact, it's possible your erections will
get worse, you may lose feeling in the penis or it might feel differ-

ently, there could be an injury to the urine channel called the urethra, you could have scarring or a change in the appearance of the penis when it's either soft or erect. And as with any operation, you could have infection, bleeding, or chronic pain."

"Have any of your patients had one of those bad complications?"

"No. But that doesn't mean it couldn't happen to you. And you need to realize there's no guarantee this will work for you at all."

"I understand. Let's go for it," said Jose.

Jose's surgery went well, and I saw him back in the office two weeks later, accompanied by Rita.

"Doctor, I haven't tried to have sex yet, just like you told me, but I'm waking up with erections in the middle of the night that are harder than before!" Jose seemed very pleased.

Jose appeared to be healing nicely, and I gave him the green light to begin having sex.

Three months later he and Rita returned for a follow-up visit. "Doctor, you did it!" exclaimed Jose, shaking my hand vigorously. "I'm back!"

"I like good news," I said. "Tell me about it."

"My erection is like old times. It gets hard and stays hard. Rita and I have been wearing this thing out!" Jose winked at me and then looked over at Rita, happy as a schoolchild. "It's like having a new toy."

"Rita, what are things like for you now?" I asked.

"It's good," she replied. "Jose is happier, that's for sure. He'll tap me on the shoulder in bed in the morning when I still want to sleep, saying, 'Honey, wake up! Look at this hard thing I found! Touch it, touch it!' " Rita and Jose laughed. She then asked, "Why are men so obsessed with their dicks?" and Jose again burst into laughter.

"Rita, now *that* is a great question," I replied. "Why do *you* think men are obsessed with it?" I asked her.

She didn't hesitate. "I think men see their penis as an extension of themselves. Well, I know it *is* part of them, obviously it's part of their body, but that's not what I mean. What I mean is they *are* their penis!" Rita had more to say. "When Jose's penis was soft, it was like Jose himself became soft. Now that his penis works again like before, he's his old self again. Fun, confident, secure in who he is."

I looked over at Jose to see his reaction. "I don't have any idea what she's talking about," he said with a comedic shrug of his shoulders. "I'm just glad it works again."

Jose did well for six months. Then he noticed that his erections weren't staying firm quite as long. By ten months he was back to where he'd been prior to surgery. His leak had returned. Jose was disappointed but decided to try penile injections to help with his erections.

"Sex is pretty good," Jose said when he returned for follow-up two months later. "It's still a little weird to take the needle when I want to have sex, but you were right, it doesn't hurt at all. It's more of a mental thing. Rita's happy, and I'm okay with it."

No Feeling, No Problem

Duncan was a twenty-seven-year-old paraplegic who had injured himself four years earlier diving into a quarry with some friends after a few beers. He wheeled himself breezily into the exam room, wearing a T-shirt cut so as to reveal a heavily muscled chest and arms. His skinny, useless legs were strapped to the lower part of the wheelchair. "Doctor, I heard there is a type of medicine I can inject to give me a hard-on. Is that right?"

Duncan had married his rehabilitation nurse, Janet, two years earlier, but they'd been unable to have "normal" sex. His spinal cord injury had left him paralyzed below the waist. In addition, he had no sensation in his legs and in his genital region. Erections were rare, fleeting, and unrelated to sexual thoughts or stimulation. They happened from time to time when he moved into or out of his sleek, high-tech wheelchair, and sometimes when he had a bowel movement.

"How long do your erections last when you do get them?" I asked.

"Thirty seconds or so," Duncan replied. "Janet has tried to jump on me a couple of times when they've happened." He smiled a crooked but engaging smile. "But we've never succeeded in getting me inside her."

"Do the two of you do anything else sexual together?"

"Oh sure. Janet loves sex! We do a bunch of things, but obviously not the one regular thing, because my penis is dead." Duncan said this matter-of-factly, without any apparent self-pity. "Doctor, if those injections are legit, I'd really like to try them. Janet deserves it. She's a young woman with a healthy sex drive, and she's put up with my physical limitations for so long. She has a birthday coming up, and I'd sure like to surprise her."

The problem for men with nerve injuries like Duncan's is that the penis doesn't receive the brain signals indicating sexual arousal, and so the penis never begins the process to create greater blood flow into the corpora cavernosa. The brain may get turned on, but the penis has no way of knowing it. Injection therapy usually works very well in men like Duncan with spinal cord injuries. They sometimes work *too* well, resulting in an erection that can last for many hours. The medications work directly on the smooth muscle controlling erection in the corpora cavernosa, bypassing any need for a signal from the nerves.

I taught Duncan how to do the injections and sent him home with prescriptions for medicine and needles, and with instructions to see me in two months.

"How are the injections working?" I asked when he returned for his follow-up visit.

"Great!" he replied. "Omigod, that stuff is amazing! I get rock-hard, just like I did before my accident, and the erection lasts for a couple of hours. Janet hops on and won't get off of me! She can have one orgasm after another." He was happy. "Hey, remember when I first came to see you I told you that Janet had a birthday coming up? That was the first time we did it. When she came home from work I was waiting in bed. She came into the bedroom, and I pulled off the covers. My dick was standing straight up, and I had tied a red ribbon around it in a bow! Janet said that was the best birthday gift ever! I love this stuff."

"When we first met you said you had almost no sensation in your penis. What do you feel now during sex?"

"Not much."

"Are you able to have an orgasm? Can you come?"

"Nope." Duncan did not seem bothered by this at all. "I haven't come once since my accident, and at this point my rehab docs tell me they don't think I ever will. It doesn't matter." He shrugged his shoulders. "At this point sex isn't about me anyway. I can't tell you how great it is to be able to do this for Janet finally. Don't get me wrong, though. I enjoy it too. I get really into it."

"What do you mean?"

"Well, this whole sex thing. It's kinda primal, don't you think? I mean, at our root, we're all animals, and this is what animals do. They have sex. In my mind, I'm doing what I'm supposed to be doing, and that feels good, even though I don't feel a damn thing in my penis."

"That's a fascinating way of looking at it. Tell me, how often have you been injecting?"

Duncan's face reddened. "I've got to apologize to you, Doc."

"What do you mean?"

"I've been a bad boy," Duncan confessed. "I know you told me not to inject more than once or twice a week, and I've been doing it just about every single day." He brightened. "But I haven't noticed anything bad from doing it so often!"

"Why are you injecting so frequently?"

"I told you when we first met, Janet really likes sex. And I want to give it to her. I'm sorry. It's incredible to be able to please my wife so much sexually. I was pretty depressed after my accident.

It was so stupid of me to dive into the quarry. I was showing off, that's what I always did. I wasn't so sure I was glad that my buddies dragged me out of the quarry instead of letting me drown. Janet took care of me in rehab. I was there for months. She was real pretty, and I flirted with her a lot, but I felt like a joke. I had no feeling in my dick, it never got hard, and I knew I would never walk again, let alone have sex.

"Janet didn't seem to care. She was the kindest anyone had ever been to me, and it wasn't that she felt sorry for me. I never felt that. We stayed in touch after I left rehab and started dating. She's done everything a person can do to make me feel okay about myself as a human being. But I always felt incomplete, inadequate.

"I get around just fine with my chair—I can live without my legs. I still didn't feel right about myself as a husband, though, and there were plenty of times when I'd feel down and think to myself that I should just leave, so Janet could find a man who could give her what she deserved.

"Now, though, with the injections, it's a new game. I feel like Superman, sometimes, because there was no way my dick would stay hard that long in the past. There are a few paras [paraplegics] at the gym I go to, and we're all macho with each other. I know they're all dealing with the same stuff. When you feel okay about yourself as a man, you don't have to prove as much to other guys. Know what I mean?"

Duncan paused for a moment. "Janet would say the injections and the erections they give me aren't important. They're important to me, though. Even though she's the one having the orgasms, I think I'm the one who feels best after we're done. Janet teases me about it. She'll say, 'You think you're da man, don't you?' and then she squeezes my nipples so hard they hurt."

I thanked Duncan for sharing his insights with me, and I gave him some further instructions regarding the injections. When we were done, Duncan asked if he could introduce me to Janet.

Duncan wheeled himself ahead of me to the waiting room. There was Janet, a pretty young woman with long, wavy auburn hair. "Hey babe," Duncan said, greeting her. Janet leaned down to give him a quick kiss, then turned to me. "This is Dr. Morgentaler."

"Hello, Doctor. I want to thank you for everything you've done for Duncan," she said.

"It's my pleasure," I replied. "I'm glad things are working out."

"Oh, they are!" said Janet, and she and Duncan laughed. "The best part, though," she added, "is that Duncan has a spark in him I'd never seen before. He's so much happier since he came to see you. And he's nicer to me too!"

Surgical Erections

After Brindley put sexual medicine on a biological foundation, there was great excitement for biological treatments for men with ED. Injections by themselves were a remarkable advance, and the ability to perform vascular studies on men was enormously helpful in making the diagnosis and explaining to men why they were having trouble with their erections. Epidemiologic studies were being done to define the extent of the problem, and it quickly became apparent that ED was remarkably common, increased in prevalence as men aged, and was associated with the same risk factors that were known to be bad for blood vessels in general.

Since the penis could now be considered a specialized blood vessel, a number of investigators around the world began exploring vascular solutions to ED. Penile venous ligation, the procedure I performed on Jose, became very popular during this time. It was a straightforward, clean operation, there were few problems with it, and many men had immediate positive results. Eventually, though, it became clear that in nearly all cases the venous leak returned, as it did with Jose. The real problem was that the tissues within the corpora cavernosa were impaired. Tying off some of the veins could help for a while, but eventually the blood would find a way out. Within a couple of years of Jose's procedure I had given up performing penile venous ligations altogether, as did almost all of my colleagues.

Another operation that had more promise was a bypass procedure for blocked arteries to the penis, called a penile revascularization. It worked best in young men whose arteries feeding the penis had been injured from trauma. In those cases an artery feeding the underside of the abdominal muscles was used to provide new blood to the penis, bypassing the blocked artery much like the cardiac surgeons do in a coronary bypass operation. I had quite a few long-term successes with that procedure. However, there were few good candidates, and once Viagra became available the operation seemed like a long slide for a short gain. Today, only a handful of surgeons continue to offer penile revascularization, but it can be a good option for a highly selected group of young men.

9. THE BIONIC PENIS

The Penis Bone

Problems with erections have been with us forever, and men have been trying to find solutions for just as long. For centuries, men had tried one way or another to augment their own erections by strapping various materials to the penis. Some men have shown me photos of their homemade products, most of which apply something like Popsicle sticks to the outside of the penis to act as a stiffener.

Early surgical ideas took inspiration from the animal kingdom. Quite a few mammals, including the dog and raccoon, have a bone in the penis, called the *os penis* (Latin for "penis bone") to help with the tricky business of inserting the penis into the vagina. The walrus is credited with the largest *os penis*, called an oosik by native Alaskans. In 2007, there was an auction to purchase a 4.5-foot-long fossilized oosik from a larger and now extinct animal in the walrus family. Oosiks from walruses, seals, or polar bears are polished and used as knife handles or carved and sold to tourists. Several of the apes have an *os penis*, too, but alas, through the wisdom or shortsightedness of evolution, humans have lost this potentially useful sex aid.

Aware of this human anatomic deficiency, surgeons thought it might be useful to correct Nature's oversight. In the middle of the twentieth century a number of procedures were performed to place stiffeners under the skin of the penis. One of these was rib cartilage. The concept seemed solid enough, but the results were not. The cartilage tended to move around, causing discomfort and inadequate support. Moreover, the cartilage was soon degraded and absorbed by the body, leaving only useless scar tissue behind. Later attempts involved insertion of plastic or similar materials that could not be degraded, often combined with techniques to anchor them to the pubic bone to provide more support. The results were not particularly satisfactory, and by all reports, the penis looked and felt strange.

The big conceptual advance was to place something deeper inside the penis, into the corpora cavernosa. The first devices, made from a firm latex rubber, worked well but were so firm that the men with these early implants walked around with a perpetual erection. This was unacceptable, especially in the prim 1950s. Later versions of these solid implants had some give, so the penis could be worn partially downward during the day, but there were still issues of concealability.

During my residency in the mid-1980s it was routine to instruct men who received these semirigid implants to wear snug underwear in combination with loose trousers, and to avoid light-colored materials, so that the penis wouldn't be too obvious. Ad campaigns in medical journals for competing models proudly reported the angle at which the penis could be bent downward, and how well the devices managed the problem of "springback." Modern versions of these implants have largely solved the concealability and springback issues. Men who have one of these noninflatable penile implants now walk around with the penis pointing downward, and when they want to have sex they simply take the penis and point it upward and outward, as if adjusting a goose-neck lamp.

These malleable, solid implants are fine—they provide a firm erection, are easy to implant, and are extremely durable. However, most men would prefer a device that allows their penis to get hard and soft, as their own penis used to do, and today most implants are of the inflatable type.

Shock and Awe

When I was younger, with a more limber back, I was an avid and reasonably accomplished squash player. During residency I gave it up, but later returned to the game and joined for a time the venerable Boston Tennis and Racquet Club. The club was founded in 1902 and claims to be the oldest athletic and social club in Boston.

One Tuesday evening after a squash match I sat at the club bar, decorated with paneled walls and leather chairs, and had a beer with my playing partner, Kelly, a business consultant. "Do urologists do surgery?" he asked.

"Yes," I replied. "We're a surgical specialty. Urologists do operations for prostate cancer, kidney cancer, stones. Almost any kind of surgery you can imagine for the urinary system and for 'guy stuff.'"

"Did you do any operations today?"

"Mm-hmm."

"What kind of operation?"

"I put in a penile implant."

"What?" Kelly asked incredulously. "What do you mean, *a penile implant*?"

"I put an implant in a man's penis. In fact, I did two of those today."

"Come on, you're joking. There's no such thing as an implant for the penis!"

"There is."

Kelly looked at me for a moment, deciding whether I was pulling his leg. "Why do guys get them? To make their dicks bigger?"

"No," I said, laughing. "Not for that. The implants don't make the penis any bigger. They're for men who aren't able to have an erection."

"That's amazing! You actually put something inside the penis?"

"Yes."

Kelly turned to his right and called over another squash player. "Bunky, get this. Abe, here, is a urologist, and he says that today he did an operation where he put an implant inside a man's dick!"

Bunky took a few steps toward me, Scotch in hand. He extended his hand and introduced himself. "This guy you operated on must have had a tiny piece of equipment, right? Like Kelly," he said, winking at me and nodding his head toward his friend.

"Actually, the implants don't make anyone bigger. They're not like breast implants. They help guys who can't get hard anymore."

"Why not just use Viagra or Cialis?" asked Kelly.

"The pills don't always work," I explained.

Bunky called over a few folks at the other side of the small room. In a moment I was surrounded by about six men and a couple of women too. "Do you really put something inside a man's penis?" asked one of the women. "What's it made of?"

I was smiling. The group was hanging on my every word. "The implant is made of silicone. It's like a soft plastic."

"How does it work?" asked another man in the crowd.

"There are two hollow tubes that go inside the two chambers of the penis that normally produce the erection, and they're filled with saline, or salt water. There's a pump that sits in the scrotum, like a third testicle. When the man wants to have sex, he finds the pump in his sac, gives it a few squeezes, and the penis goes up."

"He'd better not squeeze the wrong thing down there!" joked one of the men.

"Yeeeoowww!" said another, and pantomimed the painful response to squeezing a testicle.

Kelly was entranced. "Does it hurt when the guy pumps it up?" he asked. "And can he still come?"

"Once he heals up, there's no discomfort involved at all," I explained. "And everything else works normally: sensation, ejaculation, urination. The only thing wrong with these guys is that there's a problem with their hydraulic system, so they can't get hard. The implant solves that problem. All the other systems work the same as before, but now they can have a hard penis when they want to."

"It feels just as good when a man comes?" asked Kelly.

"Yup," I answered. "Same as before. Sometimes better, because it's easier to get the right kind of stimulation when the penis is good and hard."

The second woman in the group had been listening to me with her hand over her mouth, wide-eyed. "I've never heard of such a thing," she said. "What's it feel like for women?"

"The women say it feels normal," I answered. "My colleagues and I have published a couple of medical articles on this, and about ninety percent of the female partners of men with implants say they're happy."

"It doesn't feel weird when they have sex?" she persisted, not quite believing me.

"Believe it or not, I had one patient come to the office recently who has remarried since I put in his implant six years ago, and he tells me his new wife doesn't even know he has one!"

"Must be one of those women who are afraid to go near a guy's stuff," said Bunky.

"She's a nurse," I said.

"Yeah, right," said Bunky, disbelievingly.

"It's true," I replied.

"Are you saying there's no way a woman can tell if a man has an implant?" asked the first woman.

"No, of course she can," I replied. "It's more difficult to tell when the device is inflated, because the penis does become hard just the way it should, all along the shaft. When it's soft, though, you can feel parts of the implant within the penis or in the scrotum that don't belong there, but you'd have to be really feeling for it."

"There's no plastic or anything that sticks out?" asked Kelly.

"No," I answered. "In fact, you guys have probably showered with someone here at the club who has an implant, and you'd never know."

"I knew it!" exclaimed Bunky. "Kelly, why didn't you just tell us you were a patient of Abe's?" he said, slapping him on the back.

The Tuesday Special

Just about every Tuesday for over twenty years I've placed one or more of these implants in men. They are by no means rare, but for some reason the penile implant remains almost unknown. Perhaps it's because the implants don't show in men, unlike a woman with new breast implants whose clothes suddenly fit her differently. Perhaps it's because men who get an implant feel shame for having ED in the first place and never mention it to anyone. And perhaps it is because penile implants in men are so much less common than breast implants in women. Every year there are only about 14,000 operations for penile implants in the United States, compared with over 250,000 breast implants in women.

The implants are often considered a last resort for men with ED, but if so, they are a marvelous last resort. Men with implants are some of my happiest patients ever. Nearly all men with ED will first try pills, and if those don't work many will move on to injections. However, the injections also don't always work, and many simply can't get used to the idea of giving themselves a shot in the penis, even though the injection itself is almost painless. Other choices exist for the treatment of ED, like vacuum pumps and a tiny suppository called MUSE that goes into the urethral opening, but these are not widely used due to limited efficacy or lack of appeal. In contrast, the beauty of the implant is that it definitely, absolutely solves the ED problem. And once healed, the penis looks normal, feels normal, and sex is easy. There's no need to plan ahead, as with the pills, or to psych oneself up for an injection. All it takes is ten to twenty seconds to give the pump a few squeezes, and then it's time for "Honey! Look what I've got!"

The implants also provide a unique perspective on male sexuality, since they allow a man to have sex anytime, anywhere, and for as long as he likes, whether or not he's aroused. When Viagra was first introduced, a commonly heard fear among women was that the medication would make their partners sex-crazed due to their newfound sexual prowess, and they would then leave their spouses for younger women or have affairs with anything in a skirt. If that were true for men with Viagra, consider how much easier it would be for men "to go crazy" with an implant. This concern that men with a firm erection—whether natural, pharmacologically enhanced, or mechanical—would engage in nonstop sex presupposes that men dictate when sexual relations occur. To which nearly any man in my practice would say, "Ah, if only that were true!"

Take Grady, for example. Grady was a forty-seven-year-old plumber who came to see me a year after his implant surgery. All was going well, he said, and he was pleased with the implant.

"How often are you having sex?" I asked.

"Only about once every two to three weeks," he replied.

"Would you like to have sex more frequently?"

"Sure! Who wouldn't?"

"So what's stopping you?"

Grady shrugged his shoulders in response, as if he didn't really know.

"Well, is it you who initiates sex usually? Or your wife?" I probed, trying to be helpful.

"Doctor, I *initiate* all the time," he said, poking fun at my technical lingo, "but my wife, Doreen, doesn't let me *consummate*! She has to be in just the right mood for anything to happen. Kids have to be fed and asleep, laundry has to be done, dishes cleaned, no early appointments the next day. The list goes on and on." Nearly all of my patients will say that it is the woman who determines when sex will take place, whether or not a man is able to have an instantaneous, bionic erection.

I did have one patient whose implant changed how often he and his wife had sex. Josh was twenty-seven years old and had suffered a pelvic injury at his construction job, causing damage to his bladder and damaging the deep tissues of the penis, rendering him nearly completely impotent. He underwent surgery to repair his bladder and had plates placed to stabilize his pelvis, but his erections never returned. The pills didn't work, and Josh decided he was too young to be injecting his penis every time he wanted to have sex. Josh was married to Kate, an administrative assistant at an auto supply firm, and they had a three-year-old son, conceived before Josh's injury. Josh had the implant surgery with me and did well. One day I received a phone call from Kate, about two weeks after I'd given Josh the green light to start having sex again.

"Doctor, something is wrong with Josh," she said.

"What's the problem?" I asked.

"He doesn't come anymore during sex. You must have cut something at surgery, a nerve maybe. He gets hard and all, but he doesn't come."

This was an unusual and potentially serious problem. However, it didn't make much sense. Damage to the sensory nerves of the penis can certainly result in difficulty achieving an orgasm, but it was almost inconceivable that Josh's nerves could have been injured at surgery since the sensory nerves run along the top surface of the penis, and all the work to place the implant had been performed via the underside of the penis. Yet Josh had experienced major trauma to the nearby area and had undergone reconstructive surgery. Perhaps his anatomy had been altered by one or both of those events. "Kate, has Josh ever been able to come since the surgery?" I asked.

"Yes," she said, to my great relief. "But it's not every time anymore. Maybe one out of three times we have sex. That's not right."

"Kate, how often are you and Josh having sex?" I asked.

"Well, that's the other thing I wanted to talk to you about. Ever since you told him it was okay to have sex again, he's been like a madman. He's after me all the time. Before we get out of bed, after I shower, after breakfast, as soon as I come home from work. I'd say we're doing it five or six times a day now. Is there something about the implant that makes a man horny like that?"

Kate told me she hadn't discussed any of this with Josh yet. She'd wanted to check in with me first. I reassured Kate as best I could and told her I wanted to see Josh in the office.

He came in two days later, strutting like a rooster. I shared with him what Kate had told me.

"Wow. I'm sorry Kate bothered you, Doc. Everything is fine," Josh reported.

"Kate seemed surprised you don't have an ejaculation every time you have sex," I said. "Are you bothered by that too?"

"Not really. Of course it would be nice if I could come every time, but I realize I'm not fifteen anymore. We're having a lot of sex, Doc," he explained proudly. "I'm lucky if I can come two or three times in one day, and we're doing it more often than that."

"That's the other thing Kate mentioned. She said she thinks you've gone crazy with sex."

Josh got red in the face when I mentioned this. "She said that?"

"Yes. What's that all about?"

Josh didn't answer right away. When he did, it was in a more subdued voice. The cockiness was gone. "Doc, I can't begin to tell you how bad I felt when my penis didn't work. There I was, a young guy with a young, beautiful wife, and my dick was as dead as a doorknob. I recovered fine from my accident and then the surgery, and everyone told me how good I looked. That was all on the outside, though. Inside, I was a mess. I felt like a fake.

"I felt sorry for myself. But the person I really felt sorry for was Kate. She'd been through my whole recovery, she took care of our kid, and she was supporting us, really, because I couldn't work. Even when I recovered, I still couldn't give her sex. So when you told me I could go for it again after the operation, that's what I did. Making up to Kate for all the lost time, I guess." Josh shook his head, upset with himself. "I hadn't really thought about it much, but I hear myself now, and I sound like an idiot. Somehow I thought I needed to prove to Kate that I was really back, and she could count on me again for sex."

I wanted to get back to the orgasm issue. "Josh, when you're having sex five or six times a day with Kate, do you feel hungry for sex each time you do it?"

"You mean am I horny every time?" he asked. "Nah, not really," he admitted with a wry smile. "I think that's part of the reason I don't always come."

Josh didn't have a nerve injury. Rather, he'd had an injury to the male ego, that part of himself that felt he needed to prove to his wife that he was a sexually capable man. In his mind, young, healthy men should be having sex as much as they possibly could. And now that he had a device he could pump up anytime, whether or not he was in the mood for sex, he was acting out what he thought he needed to or should do. The implant allowed him to have sex even when he lacked the desire. In the history of mankind, this possibility had never before existed.

"Josh, I think Kate will be *relieved* if you cut back a bit on the sex," I said.

Josh smiled. "I bet you're right, Doc. I've been wearing us both out." And then, half serious, he asked, "Are all the men you see as dumb as me?"

"You're not dumb, Josh," I replied seriously. "It's hard to always know the 'right' way to act, especially when it comes to sex. So guys improvise, and sometimes what they come up with can be a bit odd, despite their best intentions. Don't beat yourself up, though. No harm done. You have a wife who loves you, and you've had a full recovery from the accident. You're a lucky man."

In the Operating Room

It was another Tuesday, and as usual I was in the operating room doing an implant case. Asleep on the operating room table was Vincent, forty-eight, who had been diagnosed with an aggressive form of prostate cancer and had undergone a radical prostatectomy a year earlier to remove the cancerous gland. The surgeon had taken as much extra tissue around the prostate as he could to reduce the chances of leaving any cancer cells behind. Unfortunately, this meant that the nerves necessary for creating erections had also been cut in order to get the wide margins on the cancer. Fortunately, at one year, Vincent's blood tests indicated no recurrence of his cancer, which was a very positive sign.

Vincent could become sexually excited, but his penis never even became fat. He had tried the ED pills without success. This poor result was not surprising given that the pills don't work well in men after prostate cancer surgery. The pills augment the chemical signal triggered by the nerves that run alongside the prostate. But if the nerves have been injured and can't supply a signal to begin the erection process, the pills can't make that nonexistent signal any stronger.

Vincent had success with the injections and had used them for several months with his wife, Marie, but when he celebrated his good one-year blood tests, he decided to take a more permanent approach to his sexual problem. When I'd sat in the office with the couple, Marie had indicated she wasn't sold on the idea of a penile prosthesis for Vincent.

"Doctor, I want you to know that I've told Vincent he shouldn't be doing this for me. I'm perfectly fine with how things are going right now," she told me.

"Honey," said Vincent, "are you saying you don't want me to do it at all?"

"I'm saying this is your decision," she said to him, raising both hands as if she were refusing responsibility for whatever was to follow.

In the preop holding area before surgery, Vincent said to me as he was about to be wheeled into the OR on his stretcher, "Doc, did you get a good night's sleep? I don't want you to have too much of a tremor while you're operating on the family jewels."

"I slept like a baby," I assured him.

"Good. Listen, I know Marie didn't seem too enthusiastic about my having the surgery, but she'll be all right. She's just nervous about me having surgery again."

In the OR, Vincent drifted off to sleep under the skillful care of the anesthesiologist. I made a delicate incision along the natural line going down the middle of the scrotum onto the underside of the penis. I placed small hooks along the incision, exposing the white tunica albuginea sheathing the corpora cavernosa. With electrocautery, I then opened the tunica albuginea on the right side, deep in the penis where it joined the scrotum, and the spongy tissue of the corpora cavernosa came into view. I did the same for the left side.

Next I dilated the corpora cavernosa to make room for the implant cylinders. I took out a measuring device and passed it up and down Vincent's corpora cavernosa. The length was twenty centimeters, approximately eight inches.

Now most men with an eight-inch penis would feel like a king, but remember that this measurement included the part of the penis we don't see that travels under the scrotum. From his pubic bone to the tip of the penis, Vincent's penis on full stretch was still a respectable five and a half inches. I placed the cylinders into the opened corpora cavernosa and then sutured the tunica albuginea over the cylinders to enclose them inside. At the bottom of the incision, narrow tubing exited each side, joining in the middle at a teardrop-shaped pump, about the size of a squat, rounded memory stick. I placed the pump low in the scrotum where it could be easily grasped below and slightly behind the testicles. Before closing the skin, I had the resident assisting me, Yuri, inflate the device. He gave it four quick pumps, and the penis stood up straight.

"What do you think?" I asked Yuri.

This was the point in the operation when everyone stopped

what they were doing to take a look. The female anesthesiologist looked over the top of the drapes to see Philip's penis standing up. The scrub nurse stopped counting sponges to look. The circulating nurse hung up the phone and walked over to the operating table. And the female medical student, Arabella, on her first day of surgery rotation, stood across from me, eyes wide.

Yuri examined the penis carefully, feeling that the tips of the two cylinders were equal in length and supported the head of the penis. He squeezed the sides of the penis to assess the rigidity. "Seems good to me," he said.

"Watch," I said. "It is important to see how firm it is in an axial direction," pushing down a bit on the tip of the penis, seeing if it would buckle. "The key to rigidity is to be able to penetrate the vagina, to get inside."

Yuri pushed down as I'd shown him. "Got it. This thing is *firm*. It will never buckle," he said, admiringly.

"Looks good to me," said the circulating nurse.

"To me too," the anesthesiologist agreed.

"Mmm-hmm," agreed the scrub nurse.

"Good," I said. "Now, Yuri, go ahead and deflate it."

Yuri bent the penis and held it bent for a count of ten, then released it. The penis softened and hung limply.

Arabella spoke up. "Dr. Morgentaler, um . . . may I . . . ?"

"You want to inflate it?" She nodded. "Go ahead. Here's the pump," I said, showing her. "Use two hands. One to hold it in place and the other to squeeze the bulb at the bottom."

She did as I instructed, and with a few pumps the penis was standing up again.

"Why don't they make these things with a remote control, instead of needing to pump it up?" asked the scrub nurse.

"It's been considered," I answered, in as serious a voice as I could manage, "but we worry about what would happen if the remote control got into the wrong hands."

"And you'd have to worry about interference from garage door openers!" added Yuri.

"I never imagined I would see something like this when I entered medical school," Arabella said.

Every Tuesday for more than twenty years I've pumped up penises and deflated them, and after all this time I am still amazed. Every single time. One of the most basic yet almost secret events in human physiology, an erection, recreated hydraulically with an artificial device. Arabella would remember this case for the rest of her life.

Vincent did well with his surgery. Four months after I'd given him permission to use the implant for sex he returned for a routine visit. Everything was fine, he told me. He and Marie were having sex about once a week, and he had no pain. "One of the interesting things for me," he said, "is that when I was using the injections I was able to have sex, but I still felt impotent. Now, with the implant, I don't feel impotent anymore. I know it's not part of me naturally, but in a strange way I feel like it is."

I reminded Vincent that Marie had been hesitant about the surgery, and asked how she felt about it now. "Doctor, you wouldn't believe it. Marie is your biggest fan. Saturday is our 'date night,' and every Saturday night when we go to sleep, Marie says, 'Bless you, Dr. Morgentaler!'"

I laughed. "What do you think changed for her?" I asked.

"I knew sex was important for Marie, despite her religious upbringing. I figured she would be happy once I made it through the operation. She was just scared for me, that's all, and didn't want to feel responsible for pushing me into it in case I had a complication."

Like Examining Melons

Walter was fifty-six years old but looked about ten years older, partly because he had a sizable belly. He also had suffered from a viral infection that had blinded him in one eye, causing it to look pale and vacant. When I learned he had made an appointment to see me, I wondered what might be wrong. I had first met Walter fourteen years earlier. When he was forty-two, I had operated on him to place a penile implant. After eleven years that device had failed, and I had replaced it with a new one. Since the average life span of the implants is about ten to twelve years, there was nothing unusual about that story. However, it was now only three years since the last surgery, and as I entered the room I was hoping that Walter's new device hadn't failed prematurely.

Sitting next to Walter was a beautiful woman in her early forties. Walter introduced us—her name was Julie. Her long auburn hair was swept up and over one side of her face and reached down below her shoulders. She wore a pair of bright, stylish glasses, smiled easily as we shook hands, and said, "It's nice to meet you" in a warm voice.

"Hi, Walter," I said. "What brings you to see me today?"

"Hi, Doctor," began Walter. "I'm here because, well, I'm not sure things are working out with the implant the way they're supposed to."

"What do you mean?"

"You know, that first implant I had, I kinda figured it broke because I wore it out. Not that I was having very much sex. I was pumping it up for myself, if you know what I mean." He raised an eyebrow, the one over his good eye, to make sure I understood he'd been using it exclusively for masturbation. I nodded. "Anyway, when you put the new one in, I was afraid to use it too much. In fact I barely touched it, until I met Julie. Now, I'm not sure it gets as hard as it should. Not as hard as the last one, anyway."

"Do you think it's broken?"

"Maybe. I don't really know." He turned to Julie. "Why don't you tell the doctor what you were wondering."

While Walter had been speaking with me, Julie had seemed totally at ease, comfortable and supportive. She touched him in encouragement as he struggled to find words, rubbed his back as he told me he wasn't sure what was going on. However, when Walter asked her to speak, she responded with "Oh, I wasn't prepared to say anything!" and the color drained instantly from her face. Julie's forehead started to glow with perspiration, and she pulled off her down vest. Julie stared at me for a moment as if she were thinking about what to say, then suddenly turned her head away from both Walter and me, her hair preventing me from seeing her face.

"Here are some tissues," I offered, placing them near her. She shook her head to indicate she didn't need them.

After a few moments of awkward silence, with Walter's hand on Julie's right shoulder, she brought her head forward again but tilted her chin into her chest, raised up her shoulders almost to her ears, and looked up at me over her glasses like a terrified child. In a high, quiet voice she said, "I don't want him," nodding ever so slightly toward Walter, "to think that any of this is his fault."

"Of course," I responded, as reassuringly as I could.

"I don't get . . ." She shook her head and started over. "I was wondering if you could explain to Walter, no, to both of us about the G-spot and the importance of deep penetration for a woman."

"Oh!" I thought to myself. I saw now that this meeting was moving in quite a different direction than I'd originally expected. "Sure," I said, a little too loudly, it seemed, after Julie's almost whisperlike question. "Those are important things for us to talk about. Let me just say, though, that you're very brave to bring this up." Julie was still barely looking at me over her glasses, shoulders high and head low. "One of the hardest things in the world is to talk about sex. But it's important, so I'm glad you're both here. I'd like very much to help you guys out." Julie's shoulders seemed to relax a bit. Walter had his hand on her right knee now.

"Just yesterday," I continued, "I had a man in my office who is in his late sixties, married for something like forty years. This man is well known for being a great communicator. That's one of his skills. Well, yesterday he told me that he and his wife haven't had sex in over two years. And when I asked what his wife's reaction to that was, he said to me, 'I really don't know. We've never discussed it. Not once. In fact, we've never talked about anything related to sex the whole time we've been married.'"

Julie was paying attention now, looking straight at me.

"Here's a guy whose career has been all about being able to communicate," I continued, "and in forty years of marriage he and his wife haven't talked once about sex! And now that they have a problem, they don't even have the language to discuss it. So trust me when I say you're brave for bringing this up.

"Female orgasms and the G-spot are a bit of a mystery for lots of folks. In fact, as many as twenty-five percent of women never experience an orgasm. Ever." I was watching Walter, and especially Julie as I spoke, trying to calibrate my words based on their body language. "I want to answer your questions, Julie, but may I ask you something first?" Julie nodded quietly, her head tilting a bit down again. "Are you able to have an orgasm?"

"Yes," she answered in that same little girl's voice. "Sometimes. Not lately. Not always with the penis inside. Unless it's in very deep. And Walter's penis falls out a lot when we have sex."

Aah! *This* was the reason Walter and Julie had come to see me. "I understand," I said. "Well, here's the story: People talk about the G-spot like it's a specific structure or location, but that's too technical. I think it's easier to think about the G-spot as the trigger point for women, the place that if stimulated properly makes them feel like they want to come. Different women have different trigger points. Men have something like a G-spot too. The importance of the trigger spot is recognizing that not all parts of the genital region are equally sensitive. For some folks, it is only a specific location or even a specific way to stimulate that area that actually brings a person to an orgasm."

I thought I was doing a good job explaining things, but Julie looked at me as if she wasn't getting it. Walter's expression was blank. I decided to try a more anatomical approach.

"Technically, the G-spot for women is a couple of inches inside the vagina, on the upper surface. There are a lot of nerve endings concentrated there." Julie looked at me with an expression I could only interpret as disappointment. I rambled on. "Curiously, some women don't find the actual G-spot to be their trigger. Some women, and I'm wondering if this may apply to you, Julie, get the most pleasure from deep penetration. This can be from the head of the penis hitting the cervix, something called cervical tapping."

Julie's expression softened. I was making headway, but I wasn't getting any real input from either Julie or Walter. It was time for me to shift gears.

"Walter, let's see what's going on with your implant. May I examine you?"

Walter stood up. "Of course." Julie gathered her things. "Should Julie stay or leave?"

"That's entirely up to you," I answered.

"Honey, why don't you stay," Walter suggested, and Julie sat back in her chair.

As Walter unfastened his belt, I asked casually, "So how long have you guys been together?"

"Two months," said Walter. I hadn't expected to hear they'd been together such a short time based on how familiar they seemed with each other. Just making this appointment together was an indication of a strong bond, one that usually takes longer to develop.

Walter dropped his pants. His abdomen protruded out from his body, obscuring his view of his penis from above. I could tell immediately from the way the penis hung that the implant wasn't fully deflated. I put on a pair of gloves and examined Walter. I inflated the device and then let it down again. It worked perfectly. "Walter, let's see you inflate the device," I said.

Walter started squeezing on the pump lying under the skin, in the middle of his scrotum. He squeezed too rapidly and without much pressure. The penis stood up, but it wasn't very firm.

"That's what it is, Doctor. See? It's not that hard. I can bend it almost in half."

Walter took his hands away, and I gave the device a few more pumps. The penis became much firmer. It was now a great erection. "Walter, feel it now," I said.

"Hey, that's much better!" he said. "What did you do to fix it?"

"The implant works fine. It doesn't need any fixing. You just need to take more time with each pump and squeeze it harder each time. If you can pump it up like this, I think you guys will be fine."

I deflated the implant and instructed Walter to pump it up the way I'd explained. The penis lifted up and became very firm.

"I think I was afraid of overpumping it," said Walter. "Can a guy break it by squeezing too hard?"

"No," I answered. "The firmness in the penis depends on how hard you squeeze the pump. When you can't squeeze anymore, you're done. You can't break it by overpumping."

Walter was standing with his pants and underpants around his ankles, just a couple of steps from Julie. He turned toward Julie and shuffled over to her. "Here, honey," he said. "You feel it. What do you think?"

Julie reached over and felt Walter's penis. She gave it a squeeze this way and that, as if she were examining melons at Whole Foods. I experienced a moment of awkwardness and thought that perhaps it would be better if Walter and Julie saved this for when they were home alone. Then I gave myself a swift mental kick in the shins. It was definitely odd to be in a room where a woman was feeling a man's erect penis, but there was nothing wrong with Julie feeling Walter's penis at that moment. It was about sex, of course, but they weren't *having* sex. After all these years working with couples and sex, I still got embarrassed when faced with it. Sex is the most intimate, most *private* part of our lives. It was no wonder a seemingly confident woman like Julie could be reduced to a childish voice and manner when discussing her sexual concerns.

"Your penis is definitely harder now," Julie concluded eventually. "The doctor is right. If you can get it this hard, I think sex will be much better. You were falling out before because it wasn't pumped up all the way." Julie was speaking like a grown-up now, no longer with a little girl's voice.

I instructed Walter to practice inflating and deflating his penis until he was comfortable that he could get it as firm as I had, and he then pulled up his pants.

We were one step closer to a solution, but I believed there was another problem. Although I have spent a great deal of time over my career counseling men that penis size is largely unrelated to being a satisfying partner, there are some exceptions. Some women do require particularly deep penetration to achieve an orgasm, and I wondered from Julie's few comments whether she might be one of them. If so, I wasn't worried so much about Walter's actual penis size but more by his most prominent anatomic feature: his impressively protuberant midsection.

"Walter, another thing I've noticed is that your belly may be getting in the way of sex."

"I know I need to lose some weight, Doctor," Walter said apologetically.

"You do, Walter. I know it's hard, but I have a great incentive for you now. If you lose weight, I can guarantee that Julie will enjoy sex with you more." Julie smiled at this comment, and Walter was paying close attention. "Losing weight will be healthier for you, but that's not why I'm bringing it up. The real benefit will be that you will be able to thrust deeper into Julie. If a man, or a woman, has a big belly, it's like putting a beach ball between the two of you. If you're facing each other like two parallel lines, your belly makes it tough for the penis to even reach the vagina, let alone penetrate to its full length." Julie was nodding throughout this little dissertation.

"Okay, I'm going to start today!" said Walter.

Julie turned and smiled at him, taken by his enthusiasm.

"Good!" I said. "But it takes time, and you have to keep after it. In the meantime, I have a couple of ideas for the two of you. When you're having sex, position your bodies so you're more like the letter

V. That way, the penis and vagina are able to get closer to each other without the belly getting in the way. Try doing it on your side. Or put a pillow under Julie's bottom. Or have Julie be on top—the belly flattens out when we're on our backs."

"I was thinking it might work well from behind too," suggested Julie.

"That should work too," I said. "Listen, have *fun* with this!"

Julie and Walter looked at each other hopefully, happily.

"Okay," I said, wrapping things up. "You guys both have homework to do. Walter, your job is to practice inflating the penis fully. I want you to do it every day for the next two weeks, whether or not you plan to have sex. If you have any problems, you come back to see me. And Julie, your assignment is to show Walter what feels good for you. Don't be shy. He's eager to do it." Walter nodded his head in agreement. "When you're in bed together, take Walter's hand and show him where to touch you and how to do it. When his penis is in the right spot, tell him. Guide him. All he really wants is to be able to please you, and it will be a lot easier if you helped him." Julie nodded.

Walter put his arm around Julie, pulled her close to him, and kissed her on the side of her head. She turned to face him, eyes moist, looking relieved, happy, in love. It was the kind of moment that in a movie, would seem unreal—too "sappy." Yet there it was.

I take away two valuable lessons from my experiences with men with implants. One is that armed with an automatic, mechanical erection, men don't really seem to behave much differently than with a regularly functioning penis. The implant, like Viagra on steroids, provides men with the opportunity to do whatever sexual hanky-panky they want to, limited only by their sense of what is right and their aerobic exercise capacity. To my knowledge, I have never had a patient undergo surgery for a penile implant and go over to the dark side, breaking hearts or becoming a gigolo because of his new sexual abilities.

The greater lesson, though, is how closely a man's sense of self is derived from his perceived success as a sexual provider with a woman he cares about. Today in my office I heard nearly identical comments from two men at totally different points in life and with two different issues. One was a thirty-eight-year-old man with premature ejaculation, and the other was a very fit eighty-two-year-old man with an implant who cannot achieve an orgasm during sex with his sixty-two-year-old wife. In almost the same words, as if they'd rehearsed it together, both said, "The pleasure I get from sex is from knowing that I'm giving pleasure to my partner." The older gentleman made this comment as he explained why he wasn't more upset about not being able to have an orgasm during sex (he was able to masturbate to orgasm), and the young man made the comment to explain the depths of the shame he felt at his inability to be an adequate sexual partner for his wife. His own pleasure at having an orgasm was meaningless when it occurred so quickly that his wife had no time to come as well.

10. MALE MENOPAUSE

Old age isn't a battle. It is a massacre.

—PHILIP ROTH, from his novel *Everyman*

One of the fastest-growing areas in medicine today is the use of testosterone in men, particularly during the middle years. Most of my academic credentials within medicine come from my work with testosterone, as I was one of the first to recognize that healthy men can experience an age-related natural decline in hormones that affects their sexuality and vitality, and which can be treated successfully with testosterone therapy. Just like menopause in women. Although testosterone has been used since the 1930s, it was a small backwater in medicine until the last twenty years or so. I feel as if I was there at its modern-era birth and have taken a degree of uncertain pride as I've watched the field expand. Although I've published many articles on the benefits of testosterone, my greatest contribution has been to show that the long-held belief that testosterone is risky for prostate cancer is false. As the fear of testosterone has declined, physicians have become more comfortable with it, leading to a crescendo of interest in its use.

So much of male sexuality is affected by testosterone. The stories of men who have lost testosterone and then regained it via treatment provide a critical window into the minds of men.

How William Got His Mojo Back

William was a fifty-six-year-old married accountant who came to see me accompanied by his wife, Suzette, fifty-three. "Doctor, I made this appointment for Will," Suzette said. She was a pretty brunette, perky, and brimming with energy. She wore a tight peach top and skinny jeans, showing off her trim figure. "Two years ago I got on a health kick and started seeing an integrative medicine doctor. My hormones were all out of whack. I had stopped taking estrogen on the recommendation of my gynecologist when that study came out saying hormones were dangerous for women. My new doctor says those concerns were blown way out of proportion, and I believe him, so I went back on. I feel great now. The best ever! Our kids are grown, and Will has done all right financially. These should be our best years ever. The problem is that while I'm experiencing a second youth, Will has been slipping into old age."

Suzette continued while William sat quietly next to her. "Will and I have had a lot of fun over the years. For an accountant, he was pretty wild." I looked over at William. Although there were only sparse remnants of white hair on the top of his head, his hair was long, and the ample hair at his temples was gathered behind into a short pony tail. A white square of a soul patch appeared below his lower lip—not your typical accountant. "Not anymore, though. My libido is the strongest it's ever been, and his is zilch. I want to go out in the evening, and he just wants to lie around watching TV. Will has gotten old before his time.

"Dr. Morgentaler, I read about you and your work in Suzanne Somers's book. I'd like you to see if Will can benefit from the same kind of hormone treatment I'm on. I'm not saying he should take *estrogen*. Whatever is right for a man." Suzanne Somers has been kind to mention my work with testosterone therapy in two of her books regarding men and aging, devoting an entire chapter to it in her latest book, *Bombshell*. Somers's best sellers on healthy aging have contributed to a lot of women taking hormones in the time around and after menopause. Many of those women have felt much better on hormone replacement, which prompted them to get their male partners to see me.

"William, what are your thoughts?" I asked.

"It sounds good to me, Doctor." William had a deep, resonant voice that would have sounded great on the radio. "I've got to tell you, I don't really feel bad. I just don't feel great. I feel flat, mainly. Can't remember the last time I had a belly laugh."

"And Will was always laughing!" interjected Suzette.

"I went to my own primary care doc," continued William. "He did a bunch of tests, said everything came back okay. He thinks I'm going through a phase of life. Says I might even be a little depressed. He calls it dysthymia. Not quite depression but on the way to depression. We're talking about trying an antidepressant to 'happy' me up."

William's symptoms were suggestive of low levels of testosterone, and I went through my low testosterone symptom checklist with him.

"How's your desire for sex?" I began.

"Way down," William answered.

"How often are the two of you having sex these days?" I asked.

"Not often," replied Will. Suzette nodded.

"How often is that?" I asked. William shrugged his shoulders as if he weren't sure how to answer. "Once a week, once a month, once a year?" I offered.

"It hasn't happened in at least two to three months," said William. Suzette nodded again, in confirmation.

"Are your erections hard enough to have sex when you do try? Penis inside vagina?"

"They're not the same as they once were, but they're all right. I just don't get them very often anymore."

"Do you ever wake up with erections in the morning?"

"Not anymore."

"Any trouble having an orgasm? Does it take more time, more work?"

"I don't think so."

"Honey," said Suzette gently, "it's definitely taking longer. Don't you remember on our trip to Belize last year you couldn't even come?"

"Yeah, but I think that was just because I was tired," said William. Then, turning to me: "Maybe she's right. It might take longer."

"What about the intensity of the orgasm? Does it still feel amazing?" I asked.

William seemed to be a bit uncomfortable with this question. He hesitated before answering, "Amazing? No, not amazing. It feels good, of course, but not like it used to be."

"I'm sorry to ask such personal questions," I said. "The reason is that I'm wondering if you do have low levels of hormones as Suzette suggested, specifically, low levels of testosterone. If you do have low T, as I like to call it, it can cause a wide variety of symptoms, and I'd like to know which ones are affecting you. No one has *all* the symptoms, but the more that are present, the more likely it is that a man has the condition. The good news is that low T is easily treatable, so if you've got it, it's worth knowing about it. When a man's testosterone levels drop, which usually happens because of age, the changes he experiences are physical. I don't know yet for sure that you have low T, but if you do, it would explain a lot. If a guy has low T, the sexual urge just isn't there like it used to be. I had a man with low T in my office last week who told me that he wouldn't be interested in sex even if Angelina Jolie slipped into his bed naked."

"That's because she's a tramp," said Suzette.

"Sorry, she's hot," corrected William. "Besides, that's not the doctor's point."

"I get it," said Suzette.

After this exchange, I continued my checklist of questions.

"Is there less fluid when you ejaculate?"

"Definitely."

"Do you feel less sensitive in the genital region—penis, scrotum? Feel like there's less sexual electricity down there?"

"Yes."

"Okay, let's move away from sex for now. How's your energy level these days?"

"Way down."

"Do you feel more tired than you think you should?"

"Yes." William exhaled deeply.

"What about motivation? Motivation to do extra projects at work, to exercise, to do projects around the house?"

"I don't do *anything* anymore. Suzette is right about that. That's why my regular doc thought I might be depressed."

"Let's talk about this depression thing, William. What is your mood like these days?"

"Like I said, I'm flat. Nothing excites me. Nothing seems funny. Everything is muted. I barely smile at things that would have cracked me up before."

"Are you sad? Blue?"

"No, I wouldn't say so."

"Individuals with true major depression often feel helpless, hopeless, worthless. Do you feel like that?"

"No. That doesn't describe me at all."

"What about irritability? Are you more short-tempered than before? Cranky?"

"No," William said.

"Whoa!" exclaimed Suzette. "Will, baby, come on! We've talked about this. Remember when you exploded at the kids for no good reason when they came over for dinner last week? Doctor, he's definitely more irritable. If he were one of the Seven Dwarfs, his name would be Grumpy!"

"Well, I'm not aware of it," resisted William.

"What about at work?" I asked. "What would your staff say?"

William snorted, as if I'd caught him. "Okay, okay. They'd probably say the same thing as Suzette. My longtime assistant, Georgina, just told me the other day that I'd been acting like I had a pebble in my shoe, as if something were bothering me, and I was taking it out on the whole office. She told me maybe I needed a vacation."

"One of the most fascinating things I hear when men have low levels of testosterone," I said, "is that they don't necessarily feel grumpy themselves, but everyone around them seems to notice a change in their behavior, for the worse.

"Let's move on. What about muscle stuff? Do you feel as if your muscles are smaller? Are workouts as productive as before?"

"I really wouldn't know, Doc," replied William. "I don't work out anymore."

"Have you put on fat, especially around your middle?"

"Definitely. But I figured that was just because I wasn't eating right and not exercising."

I reviewed the rest of William's medical history and then excused Suzette to the waiting room while I examined him. Once we were alone, I asked, "Any urge to masturbate these days?"

"Last time was about a month ago. I didn't even have the urge, really. It was more like I felt a duty to keep the pipes open. I was curious if I could do it."

"A duty?" I echoed. "William, there are many ways men would describe an orgasm, but a duty is not a standard one. I'm sure you didn't always think of it that way, did you?"

"No, I guess not," he replied. "Something has definitely changed."

There wasn't much to report on William's examination except for carrying about thirty extra pounds, mainly in his gut. I ordered blood tests and arranged to have William return in a couple of weeks to go over the results. He came back accompanied again by Suzette.

"What did the tests show?" asked William.

"Good news," I said. "Well, good news in the sense that there's something we can treat. Your testosterone levels are definitely low. Which means that many of the symptoms we discussed at our first meeting might improve if we bring your testosterone levels back to where they used to be, say fifteen, twenty years ago."

"Fantastic!" exclaimed Suzette. William glanced over at her, seemingly disturbed by the degree of her enthusiasm.

"How do I get treated?" he asked.

"There are three main ways," I replied. "Gels or creams that are rubbed into the skin, injections, or a pellet that's placed under the skin of the buttock. The gels are a daily treatment; you rub the stuff in after you shower. But you have to do it every single day, or else you don't get the full benefits. Injections are fine and have been around a long time, but you have to have one at least once every two weeks and ideally once a week. We can teach you to do it yourself at home. The third option is that I numb you up and place a number of pellets in your bum right here in the office. They're each the size of a grain of rice. They provide good testosterone levels for three to four months. Eventually they dissolve completely, and we do it again."

"Let's go with the pellets," decided William.

William lay down on his left side, and I cleansed the upper part of his right buttock. A pinch of local anesthetic, a tiny nick in the skin, and within ten minutes he was on his way out the door with enough testosterone under the fatty layer of his bum to keep him going with good T levels for a few months.

Three months later, William and Suzette came back to see me.

"Hey Doc, how's it going?" asked William.

"Good, William," I replied. "Thanks for asking. More important, though, how are you? I'm curious what you've noticed with the testosterone therapy."

"I'm back, Doc! I feel like myself again. Energy, mood, sex—it's all great. Suzette and I are like teenagers again!" He took Suzette's hand, sitting beside him.

"Doctor, I'd forgotten how good sex can feel. But it's not just the sex. It's like you injected me with 'Essence of William.' I'm myself, only better than I've been in years. I'm working out again too." William did look noticeably trimmer than when I'd seen him last.

"Doctor, may I say something?" said Suzette. She seemed much calmer than the last two times she'd accompanied William to my office.

"Of course," I responded.

"You've given me back my husband. It's like he was in suspended animation and woke up after a five-year sleep. We're having fun together again."

"Doctor, you know what it's like?" asked William. He was animated. "It's like in *Austin Powers* when the hero is frozen so he can survive into the future to fight the bad guy, Dr. Evil, but then Dr. Evil has someone sneak into the top-secret facility where Austin Powers is frozen, and he steals his 'mojo.' When Austin Powers wakes up, he's got no edge, no moxie. He can't fight evil anymore; he's not interested in girls. That's what I was like. It was as if someone had stolen my mojo!"

"Doctor, I hate to do this to you, but Suzette and I have to run. We have a plane to catch."

"Where are you off to?"

"Rome!" said Suzette. "That's where Will proposed to me. In front of the Trevi Fountain. Will doesn't want to call it a second honeymoon because we weren't there for our first honeymoon. But that's really what it is. Accountants can be so picky about details, you know?" She looked over at Will, beaming. "He's okay, though." Pause. "For an accountant." Suzette elbowed William in the ribs, laughing. "My funky, hunky accountant. I'm so glad I have him back."

Men Are Hormonal Too

Hormones for men? What a strange notion. Yet it's coming, like a tsunami. Over the last ten years the fastest pharmaceutical sector is testosterone, growing at more than 10 percent per year. There are a huge number of men out there who have the symptoms of low levels of testosterone. Some of them are sexual, some not. As this problem gained attention from physicians about ten to fifteen years ago, there was a push to talk about andropause, a male version of menopause.

I hated the term when I first heard it. Men aren't women, I argued. Every woman goes through menopause eventually, but not all men have symptoms of low T. Besides, men don't menstruate, so let's do away with this "pause" concept altogether. Yet as time has passed, I've come to view andropause, or male menopause if you prefer, as a reasonable way of thinking about the problem. The name still isn't right, but at least folks understand what we're talking about.

Testosterone is a tough word to say, and as I saw even the most educated of my patients stumble over the pronunciation, I started to use the term *low T* in the office and during lectures to describe the condition that has otherwise been called hypogonadism, or testosterone deficiency syndrome. My colleagues thought *low T* was too simplistic a term, but it worked for me and my patients, and I continue to use it. Nonetheless, I was surprised to hear one day that my verbal shorthand had been co-opted by the industry. Now, television and print ads ask, "Is it low T?" If I had a dollar for every time that term was used . . . Oh well.

Are Men Like Lizards?

We think of testosterone as the male sex hormone, and to a great extent this is true. However, testosterone is involved in so many biological functions for men that it is difficult to come up with a biological system that is *not* affected by testosterone. What is remarkable is that researchers have been studying testosterone in animals for many decades, yet with humans it is as if we are just beginning to learn about something brand-new.

When I graduated from my urological residency in 1988 and came on staff as a young attending physician, I was curious about testosterone because of research I had done as an undergraduate. During my training I had been taught that testosterone was important for sex drive but not much else, and that a man needed to have almost no testosterone left at all before his low T levels caused sexual issues. There was some grudging acknowledgment that perhaps testosterone treatment might help some men with erection issues, perhaps 5 percent at most, but this number was so small that no one was spending much time looking into treatments.

In my sophomore year at college, I ran into Professor David Crews, with whom I had worked on a term paper in biology the previous semester. He asked me how things were going, and I admitted I was feeling a bit aimless. That was when he invited me to work in his laboratory, and I thought to myself, "Why not?"

I started on a boring, tedious project, mapping out which parts of the lizard brain took up radioactive samples of hormones that had been previously injected into the bloodstream. In the end, the work was important and laid the foundation for more interesting research, but the daily routine was tough. After a few weeks, I was ready to politely say, "Thank you, but this isn't for me," when Professor Crews put me on a much more exciting research project.

The lizards I worked with were the American chameleon, *Anolis carolinensis*. These are the small, four- to five-inch green or brown lizards one finds in Florida and the Bahamas on trees and hotel walls. When a normal male lizard is placed in a cage with a female, the two of them go through what is called a sexual behavior, much like a dance. The male will extend the bright reddish orange flap of skin under his jaw, called a dewlap. He then does what we call a "stuttering push-up," bobbing his head up and down rapidly, as if he were a leering man saying, "Yeah, yeah, yeah." In response, the female will do a stately, single push-up, indicating she is receptive. The male will approach and repeat the behavior, extending his dewlap and performing his stuttering push-up. After a few repetitions, the male will grasp the female by the nape of her neck and mount her.

However, when the males were castrated, that is, had their testicles removed, they did none of this. They behaved as if they couldn't have cared less. Sometimes the confused female would do a push-up of her own, as if to say, "Hey buddy, I'm over here." If testosterone levels in the blood were restored in these animals, the males would again perform their usual sexual behavior. The sexual "dance" was a testosterone effect.

The exciting part of my research project was to see what would happen if I implanted hormones directly into the sexual centers in the brain. I learned to anesthetize the lizards and to bore tiny holes in their skull with a dental drill, like a neurosurgeon draining a brain hemorrhage. I designed a miniature device to deliver tiny amounts of powdered testosterone through the hole in the skull and into the parts of the lizard brain involved in sexual behavior (the anterior hypothalamus and the preoptic area).

I didn't quite know what to expect after I'd done my first testosterone insertions. The lizards lived in a large incubator that provided them with a warm, humid environment that replicated their normal habitat. For the observations, each cage was turned to the side, allowing me to see six pairs of lizards at a time through the glass doors, each with their own space, like looking at a row of apartment windows. The incubator was lit from the inside, and I sat in the dark, watching the pairs of lizards with a stopwatch and my lab book on my lap.

I had been doing the same type of observations with the castrated males prior to inserting testosterone into their brains, and it had been dull work. The males and the females would go to opposite ends of their spaces, and stay there, doing nothing for twenty minutes at a time, at which point I would remove the males and put them back in their own cages. This time it was different. Within two minutes one of the males saw the female and did his thing. His dewlap came out, and his head bobbed up and down like crazy. I couldn't believe what I was seeing. The female did her single push-up, the male repeated his behavior, and a few moments later he grasped the female with his jaw by the back of the neck and mounted her. I was nineteen years old, and this was the coolest thing I had ever witnessed.

The experiment was a home run. Castrated males behaved sexually just like normal males if testosterone was inserted in the correct parts of their brains. What this experiment proved was that testosterone is a brain hormone, and its actions on the brain are enough to organize the entire set of behavioral responses involved in male sexual behavior: attraction, behavioral display, and mating. I spent nearly three years in the lab, including every summer, and published my first three scientific papers from that experience and related experiments.

Yet during my training in medical school and residency, the testosterone story barely showed up. I did learn that testosterone was necessary for puberty in boys, and for development of what are called male secondary sexual characteristics, meaning a beard, prominent body hair, deep voice, and the Adam's apple. However, the only men for whom testosterone therapy was recommended were those who had significant medical conditions that caused them to make exceedingly low amounts of testosterone or none at all. The short list included men with Klinefelter's syndrome, a genetic disorder in which men carry an extra X chromosome, or men who had lost both testicles to trauma or cancer, or men who had surgery to remove tumors from the pituitary gland or hypothalamus in the brain, destroying the ability of the brain to send the chemical signal, luteinizing hormone (LH), to the testicles to produce testosterone.

Once I had my own practice seeing patients who had come to see me for weak erections or diminished libido, I couldn't help but wonder whether there might be a testosterone connection, given my research experience with lizards. So I started obtaining testosterone blood tests in my patients. I was immediately surprised by how many of these men had low testosterone levels. I thought it would be interesting to see whether sexual symptoms would respond to testosterone treatment, and so I asked an endocrinologist colleague how to give testosterone. She said, "It's easy. Give an injection of two hundred milligrams every four weeks."

I lined up a few cases and had my nurse inject them every four weeks, as I'd been instructed. Three months later I saw them back in the office to determine what they'd experienced with the treatment. My hope was that their erections would improve, or that their desire would increase, or both, but I really had no idea what to expect. Even if the men reported positive effects, my training had prepared me to discount some of this due to the placebo effect. What I heard, however, made a big impression on me.

One man said, "The treatment works. My erections are better. Especially for the first week or two after the injection. After that it's not so good." The next man told me, "Doctor, that stuff is incredible. My erections are better, and so is my sex drive. You didn't tell me that I would feel so much better in general, though. I've got energy to do things I haven't done in years. I finally cleaned out my garage, after three years on my to-do list." I was pleased and intrigued. However, I found his next comment curious and reminiscent of what the first man had said. "The weird thing is that the stuff only works for the first week or so. For the two weeks before my next injection, it's like you never treated me at all. It happened with each injection. I feel great for a week or two and then not so great."

When the next patient also said that the benefits disappeared by two weeks, I decided to check blood levels of testosterone. It turned out that testosterone levels went up nicely for the first ten days or so but had dropped back to their low baseline levels in all these men by fourteen days. I'd been curious about testosterone but skeptical. Yet the similar stories from each of these men told me there was something important going on, and it couldn't have been a placebo effect because it was impossible for them to have known how long the treatment would last for them. These men felt good when their testosterone was up and felt poorly again when their levels were down. Since these men, and I, had expected the treatment to last the entire four weeks, this turned out to be an accidental variation of what we call a double-blind experiment— neither the men nor the treating doctor knew this was going to happen. From that moment on, I was convinced that low T was common in men, and that testosterone therapy was truly helpful.

How Testosterone Affects Erections

A fifty-four-year-old friend came to see me after years of hearing me talk about testosterone. He wondered whether low T might be responsible for his lack of pep and his diminished interest in sex. His blood tests confirmed low levels of testosterone, and he began treatment with testosterone gel.

After a month I texted him, "How are things going with the T gel?"

"It's working," he texted back.

"Great," I responded. "What have you noticed?"

"Morning wood, baby!" he wrote back.

Testosterone acts on the brains of humans, just as it does in male lizards, and rats, and any number of species, to create sexual desire. This leads to an increased frequency of nocturnal and morning erections, which my friend found so reassuring. Testosterone controls the production of nitric oxide, the chemical signal in the penis that initiates erections. And it is also necessary for the maintenance of penile smooth muscle, responsible for the control of blood flow into and out of the corpora cavernosa.

In an experimental study in rabbits performed by my friend and colleague Abdul Traish, PhD, and his co-investigators at Boston Medical Center, castrated animals not only lost smooth muscle within the penis but also replaced some of it with fat. Fat does not belong within the corpora cavernosa.

In another rabbit experiment, Professor Traish set up a system in which he could monitor pressure within the corpora cavernosa before and after direct electrical stimulation of the nerve that controls erection. In control animals, nerve stimulation resulted in rapid development of high pressure within the penis, corresponding to a normal erection. However, in a group of animals that had previously been castrated so that their testosterone levels were reduced to zero, nerve stimulation produced only a minor increase in pressure. In a third group of animals in which testosterone had been replaced after castration, nerve stimulation again produced normal erections. Conclusion: normal erections in rabbits require the presence of testosterone. A great deal of evidence indicates that testosterone is critical for normal sexual function in men too.

If a man comes to see me with poor erections and he also has low T, my inclination is to try T therapy first rather than the Viagra-type medications. When it works, the man feels whole. His erections are better, and he often feels better in other ways too. Importantly, the man then doesn't have to take a pill every time he wants to have sex.

Researchers in Taiwan investigated the effect of testosterone therapy in thirty-two men whose erections were insufficient to go inside their partner's vagina during sex despite a full dose (100 mg) of Viagra. The men were treated with testosterone and for the next two months were asked to try to have sex *without* Viagra. If they were still unable to intromit (penetrate) at the end of the two months, they were then instructed to take Viagra in addition to their testosterone treatments. At the end of the study, one-third of the men were able to have sex just with testosterone, another third were able to have sex with the combination of testosterone and Viagra, and the remaining third were still unable to have normal intercourse. Testosterone can thus be a treatment for ED if levels are low, and can also improve the response to Viagra in many men.

"Why Am I Doing This?"

A few years after Viagra had been introduced to the market, Matthew came to see me with erectile dysfunction. In the forms he had filled out, he had listed Viagra as one of his medications.

"Does the Viagra work for you?" I asked.

"Yes," Matthew replied.

"Well, then how can I be helpful to you?"

"Doctor, the Viagra lets me *have* sex. But in the middle of doing it, I'm asking myself, 'Why am I here? Why am I doing this?' My penis is hard, but it's not like I really want to be there. It's weird. I'm hoping you can figure out what's going on with me."

Matthew's physical examination was normal. His blood tests, however, revealed low T. I treated him, and at his follow-up visit,

Matthew gave me two thumbs-up when I asked him how things were going. "I'm back to myself now," he said. "No more Viagra, Doctor. My erections are my own, I'm having sex more often, and while I'm doing it, I *know* why I'm there!"

I love that story because it underscores how odd sex really is. Two people who may not even like each other under most circumstances may still find each other physically appealing and create this strange intimacy and intermingling we call sex. What makes it all okay is our sex drive, or libido. Remove libido from the equation, though, and as Matthew discovered, sex can be a very strange experience. It still makes me laugh to think of him saying to himself, "Why am I doing this?"

A New Lease on Life

One day I received a phone call from a primary care physician whose patients included many of the most prominent families in Boston. "Abe, I've got Mr. J here. He's the big developer who's been in the news recently. He's seventy-two, his new wife is in her thirties, and he can't get it up. Viagra and Cialis haven't worked. Can you see him?"

A few days later Mr. J walked into my office. I'd read about him in the papers but had never seen a photo of him. I was surprised by his appearance when we shook hands. He was very tall, but he stood with a stooped posture and slightly bowed head. I had the urge to put my hands on his chest and back to straighten him up, as parents sometimes do with their children when they slouch. There was no way this man looked anything like a major figure in the Boston community.

"Doctor, I've gotten lucky late in life. I've been married now for a year. My wife, Mara, is the most wonderful, most beautiful woman. And I feel like an ass because I can't get it up. It's not fair to her. Those pills my doctor gave me, Viagra and the other one, they're garbage. Trying to have sex is like playing pool with a limp noodle."

"How's your desire for sex?" I asked.

"Of course I *want* to have sex," he answered. "Have you seen my wife? She's gorgeous."

"Do you have any trouble having an orgasm?"

"I wouldn't know. Haven't had one in months."

"Why not?"

"If I'm not having sex, how can I come?"

"Well, even men with weak erections can usually come if their hormone levels are all right. Do you have any urge to masturbate?"

"Nah! I haven't done that in years."

Based on his responses, I was fairly confident that Mr. J's blood tests would show low T, and sure enough they did. I started him on a gel and monitored his blood levels after a few weeks to make sure he was absorbing it at a good concentration.

Three months later, Mr. J returned to my office. He looked great, just as I would have imagined a man with his reputation and standing should look. He stood tall, his skin glowed, his eyes were bright. There was an aura of charisma and power about him. As he took his seat, I silently congratulated myself on my skill at restoring this man to his natural greatness.

"So," I asked Mr. J, with knowing confidence, "how are things going with the testosterone treatment?"

"That shit doesn't work," he said disgustedly.

I was momentarily shocked. "What do you mean, it doesn't work?" I managed to ask.

"It doesn't work," he repeated forcefully. "I still can't get it up. I've been slathering that stuff on my skin every day, like you told me to, and I still can't have sex with my wife."

"I'm sorry to hear you're still having trouble with sex. But I've got to tell you something. You do look great compared to when I saw you last."

"I know! Everyone is telling me that."

"Apart from sex, how are you feeling?"

"I do feel better since I started the testosterone. I've got a heck of a lot more energy. I've finalized two big deals at work that had been languishing for over a year. I've started working out with my personal trainer again, and I've dropped over an inch from my waistline."

Mr. J had actually done very well with T therapy, except that it hadn't solved his ED, which was the problem he'd wanted treated. I started Mr. J on a daily regimen of Cialis, which worked nicely, and he continued on testosterone therapy. Three years later he's still looking great.

Just Enough for My Wife

John was a fifty-seven-year-old school administrator who complained about nearly absent sexual desire. He appeared old-fashioned and reminded me of Mr. Rogers from the long-running children's TV show. John's testosterone levels were very low. I prescribed four pumps, the standard starting dose of testosterone gel, which he was to rub daily into his arms, shoulders, and chest. The pump is like a soap dispenser, dispensing a fixed amount of testosterone gel with each pump.

I saw John again after one month. "My sexual urges have returned," he reported with obvious delight. "I've even been nudging my wife, Diane, a little bit lately. I haven't done that in a couple of years."

A couple of months later I saw John again. "I have a confession to make, Doctor," he said, wringing his hands together. "I'm not proud of it, but I haven't followed your orders exactly."

"In what way?" I asked.

"I'm not using four pumps as you prescribed for me. I hope you're not angry."

"Not at all." It is not unusual for men to increase the number of pumps to see if they can get a better response from higher levels of T. "How many pumps are you using, then?"

"Three pumps."

"You mean three pumps on each side—right? Three on the right and three on the left, for a total of six?"

"No, Doctor. Three pumps in total."

"You're using *less* than I'd prescribed?" I asked, surprised.

"That's right, Doctor. You're not angry, are you? The treatment has been very good."

"John, I'm not angry at all. Just curious. Why are you using less?"

"It was too much for me," he replied earnestly. "When I was using four pumps, I found myself obsessed with sex. I went on the Internet to look at porn! I'd never done that in my life. I'm much happier on three pumps. I have enough desire for my wife, and that's all I want."

The Big Fear

For the last twenty years the greatest impediment to the use of testosterone therapy has been the fear that raising testosterone levels is dangerous for prostate cancer. It started with a publication in 1941 by Charles Huggins, MD, and his coauthor, Clarence Hodges, MD, in which they demonstrated for the first time that cancers can be sensitive to hormonal manipulation. These two researchers from the University of Chicago castrated men with metastatic prostate cancer and showed that levels of a chemical called acid phosphatase were reduced, indicating improvement in the cancer. This was the first treatment for advanced prostate cancer that had shown any efficacy. Within a few years, castration had become a standard treatment around the world, and Huggins, as the lead investigator, became famous, ultimately being awarded the Nobel Prize in Physiology or Medicine in 1966.

Huggins and Hodges also reported that "in all cases" the injection of testosterone to these same men with metastatic prostate cancer caused acid phosphatase levels to rise. They concluded that testosterone causes "activation" of prostate cancer and an "enhanced rate of growth." From that point forward, medical students around the world have been taught that high testosterone levels cause prostate cancer, low testosterone levels protect the prostate from cancer, and providing testosterone to a man with prostate cancer is like "pouring gasoline on a fire" or "feeding a hungry tumor."

Once I started seeing the benefits of testosterone therapy in men, my greatest concern was that the treatment I was offering might be like a pact with the devil: if these men were restored to youthful vitality and sexuality, it was at the expense of developing prostate cancer. What followed for me was a twenty-year exploration into the relationship of T and prostate cancer, eventually resulting in the widespread, albeit not yet universal, rejection of those long-standing concerns. I've written about this in detail in my book *Testosterone for Life*, but a short version of the story follows.

In the early 1990s I began performing prostate biopsies in men with low T even though they had normal levels of PSA, the blood test used to diagnose prostate cancer, since I wanted to make sure these men didn't harbor a hidden cancer in their prostates which might grow out of control if I treated them with testosterone. Although it was taught that men with low T are at extremely low risk for prostate cancer, I found an astonishingly high number of cancers in these men. In 1996 my colleagues and I published these results in the *Journal of the American Medical Association*, reporting that low T appeared to be as great a risk for prostate cancer as an elevated PSA. Low T was not protective at all.

Yet for a time I still clung to the belief that high levels of testosterone must be risky. In 2004 I published with my fellow, Ernani Rhoden, MD, from Brazil, an article for the *New England Journal of Medicine* on the risks of T therapy. After reviewing approximately two hundred medical articles, we could not find a single one that showed a compelling, worrisome relationship between high levels of T and prostate cancer. This was beyond strange. It had been universally accepted for decades that high testosterone is dangerous for prostate cancer and low T is protective, yet there appeared to be no evidence to support either of these beliefs.

To discover the source for these universally held beliefs, I made my way to the basement of the Countway Library at Harvard Medical School, which contains centuries-old medical journals. The very oldest of these are kept locked or under glass, but in the archives in the basement are volumes from the 1800s, waiting to be read by medical "archaeologists."

I found the volume holding the Huggins and Hodges article from the 1941 edition of *Cancer Research*, and as I pored over the text I had a "Eureka!" moment, like an electric buzz throughout my body. Although Huggins and Hodges had claimed that every one of their patients with metastatic prostate cancer who received testosterone developed an ominous increase in acid phosphatase concentrations, my close reading revealed they had administered testosterone to only three men. Of these, they only provided results for two. And one of these men had already been treated in another way, which made it impossible to determine the effect of testosterone alone. For the last seven decades the belief that testosterone makes prostate cancer grow like wildfire was based on results of an erratic and now abandoned blood test from a single patient!

It turns out that prostate cancer does need some testosterone to grow optimally, but it can only use a little bit. Once the need for testosterone has been satisfied by the tumor, any additional testosterone is simply excess. A good analogy is a houseplant and water. The houseplant (think prostate cancer) definitely needs water (think testosterone), but once it's been adequately watered, no matter how much additional water one gives it will not cause it to grow as tall as a sequoia tree. So it is with prostate cancer and testosterone.

Based on these findings, and despite warnings from colleagues several years ago, I started offering testosterone therapy to men with known prostate cancer. Today, men with prostate cancer fly from around the country to see me, each hoping that I will find him to be a reasonable candidate for T therapy to treat his ED. Many of them are.

In May 2011 I published with my colleagues Larry Lipshultz,

MD, and Mohit Khera, MD, from Baylor Medical College, a report in the *Journal of Urology* on thirteen men with untreated prostate cancer who received testosterone therapy for an average of two and a half years. They had an average of two sets of follow-up prostate biopsies. None of the men showed any progression of their cancers, and in 54 percent of the biopsies we couldn't find a trace of the cancer that had been there earlier. It was a small study, so we must be careful not to overstate the conclusions; however, this was the very first time since Huggins in 1941 that anyone had bothered to look directly at what actually happens to an existing localized prostate cancer when a man receives testosterone treatment. The answer appears to be: "Not much." I've since treated many more of these men, with similar, good results.

Recently, Eduardo, a wealthy fifty-three-year-old businessman from Colorado, came to see me. He had been receiving testosterone injections for his ED issues for one year, and then he was diagnosed with prostate cancer. He stopped the injections immediately, per the instructions of his various doctors, and had surgery. A month after surgery he was doing well physically, recuperating at his home in Cabo San Lucas, but psychologically he was in a funk.

"My home in Cabo is where I'm happiest," he said. "I built it when I sold my first business, and I just love it there. After the surgery, though, I felt like my world had caved in. I was depressed. My regular doctor told me it was natural to feel this way after being diagnosed with cancer, but that didn't make sense to me. I saw the cancer just like a business problem, and I'd taken care of it. No, I knew it was my low levels of testosterone. I had other symptoms too: no sex drive, and I felt tired, lazy. I knew I was in trouble, though, when I found myself watching a television show on assisted suicide and realized I was taking notes on what they used! That freaked me out. I decided to give myself a T injection that very same day. Within a few days I felt like myself again, and I've been taking the testosterone injections every week for the last month. The reason I'm here to see you is to find out if it's safe to be doing this."

I shared with Eduardo the same research stories I presented above, and I warned him there are still no large, long-term studies that definitely show that taking testosterone after prostate cancer is safe. Some men with exceedingly low testosterone levels might still be at risk for testosterone-induced growth of any remaining prostate cancer cells.

"Doctor," said Eduardo, "based on what I've experienced, I'd rather take testosterone and live well for three years than live for ten years without it."

Under my close supervision, Eduardo has now been on testosterone therapy since 2010. He has had no return of his cancer.

Crying for More Testosterone

Kyle was a forty-two-year-old former marine, now working as a regional sales manager for a pharmaceutical company. He was buff and muscular; his head had a thin patina of hair from a recent buzz cut. He came to see me with his wife, Lori, a pretty, slender blonde. They had moved to the Boston area from Oklahoma for Kyle's job.

"I was diagnosed with low testosterone a year ago," Kyle told me, "and I've been doing T injections ever since. They help, but I'm having some weird reactions. When I became a civilian I started doing some serious bodybuilding, hanging out at the gym four hours a day. I did a bunch of steroids. I knew I shouldn't have, but I did. Lori knows about it. The doctors I saw before told me the steroids poisoned my hypothalamus. I took the same stuff they use for horses, if you can believe it. When I met Lori I smartened up, but the damage was done. My sex drive was almost nil, and I had trouble with erections. Which makes no sense, right? I mean look at her!" he said, nodding toward Lori, who smiled awkwardly.

"So I had my blood levels taken, and my T was real low. The doc put me on injections. I take three hundred milligrams every three weeks. Sure helps our sex life," he said. "But I still don't feel right. Well, sometimes I do, I guess, but a lot of the time I don't. And that's why I'm here."

"What do you notice when you're not feeling right?" I asked.

Kyle looked over at Lori. "He goes through a whole personality change," she answered for him. "Some days he's the nicest guy ever. Great mood, nothing bothers him. Plays with our twins, carts them around the house, takes them to the park, and still somehow has dinner waiting when I get back from work. Then there are other days when he snaps at me for any little thing. If the kids make too much noise, he yells at me like it's my fault. I'm on eggshells around him those days."

Kyle listened to Lori respectfully, attentively. "I know what she's saying is true, Doctor. I'd be lying if I told you I knew what explained it. The other thing that's bothering me is I'm so darn emotional. We rented the animated kids' movie *Despicable Me*, and I started crying when the kids went back to the orphanage with that mean woman. Crying! Me! It's not the first time either. I was with the kids on the couch when it happened. I had to leave so they wouldn't see me all teary."

"Do you notice if those more emotional episodes happen at a particular point in the injection cycle? Say, a few days before the next injection?" I asked.

Lori and Kyle exchanged glances. "I'm not sure," replied Kyle. "Maybe."

"I'm wondering if three weeks is too long between injections for you. Nearly all men are back to their low T levels by ten to fourteen days, and in some men the testosterone levels can really bottom out after that. Let's see what happens if we put you on a weekly injection regimen at a lower dose."

Two months later Kyle and Lori returned to the office. "You did it, man," said Kyle. "I'm like a special ops force again. And I've stopped getting choked up at every little thing."

"He's been great with the kids, too," Lori added, smiling.

"That's great," I said. "People don't realize that men are hormonal too. It doesn't affect men the same way as women because

men usually don't go through the same fluctuations. But that's actually what was happening to you on your three-week cycle as your
testosterone levels would go up and down like a roller-coaster."

"Man, I've got a new appreciation for what women go
through, then!" said Kyle. "Okay, honey," he said to Lori, "no more
grief from me!"

"Yeah, right," Lori replied sarcastically. "That promise will
last all of five minutes!" she said good-naturedly.

"How are you doing with the kids' movies?" I asked.

Kyle laughed out loud. "That's still a problem, Doc! Maybe that's
just me, though, and not the hormones. The kids and I watched *Toy
Story 3* the other day, and there I was, all teary again. And then
I went online and discovered that *everyone* cries at *Toy Story 3*!"

Testosterone affects not only men's sexual desire and performance, but also their mood, thinking, muscle, fat, and sense of
vitality and well-being. When testosterone levels drop far enough,
men get suddenly sweaty and can even experience hot flashes, just
like menopausal women. Testosterone production declines with
age, but even young men can have low levels. I've treated teenagers and men in their early twenties for low T, but most men I see
with low T are in their forties and above. It's also extremely common, with some studies showing that as many as 40 percent of
men over the age of forty-five have low levels of testosterone.

Treatment is quite safe, so it's very reasonable for a man with
characteristic symptoms—low desire, weak erections, chronic
tiredness—to ask his physician to have his blood checked for low
T. Just be aware that many of the labs categorize a testosterone
result as "low" only if it is *very* low, which means that if a man has
symptoms and a T level that is at the low end of normal, it may still
be worthwhile to consider a three-month trial of treatment. As my
colleagues and I have published, men with symptoms and these
below-normal testosterone levels respond just as well to treatment as men with unquestionably low testosterone.

Since testosterone levels decline with age, some have argued this means the decline should be considered a normal part of aging and therefore should not be treated. It's an argument that we hear elsewhere: why do we have to medicalize normal aging? My response is simple. Normal aging *stinks*. Aging is associated with bad eyesight, bad hearing, bad teeth, bad joints, bad blood vessels, bad hearts, and cancer. We treat all of these in order to improve our lives and, in some cases, our longevity. Just because a condition becomes common as we age doesn't mean we should resign ourselves to it if treatment is helpful and safe.

I had exceptionally good eyesight until my early forties, at which point I found I had to hold books farther and farther away from my face in order to read them due to the "normal" age-related decline in near vision called presbyopia. Now I wear an artificial contraption of metal and plastic on the front of my face in order to read. Am I somehow disobeying the laws of nature by wearing glasses? I think not. Similarly, if a man with low T wants testosterone therapy in order to feel better and more sexual, I see no reason to deprive him of a trial of treatment just because many men his age are experiencing the same problem.

Here is a medication that can make men feel more energetic, improve erections and sexual desire, increase muscle strength and mass, decrease fat, strengthen bones, improve mood, and make men feel that their minds are sharper. Can anything really be that good? The answer is, simply, "Yes." Of course, not everyone responds to T therapy, and of those who do, the response is not always so dramatic.

As I see it, low T is underrecognized, underdiagnosed, and undertreated. In my own practice I have seen far too many men with low T who had been discouraged from trying T therapy or told they didn't even have the condition. Many of those men have responded to T therapy beautifully and feel that they are healthier, happier, in addition to being better sexually. Now that the fear of prostate cancer from T therapy is finally waning, there is no good reason to deprive men of a treatment that may help them regain their mojo.

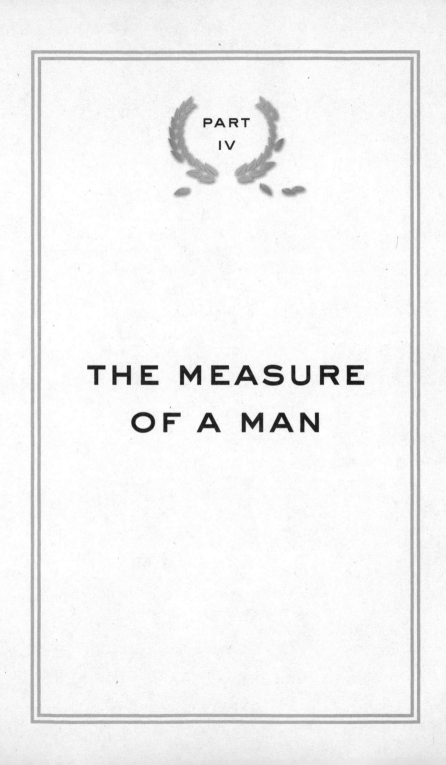

PART
IV

THE MEASURE
OF A MAN

11. AM I NORMAL?

Almost all the ideas we have about being a man or being a woman are so burdened with pain, anxiety, fear and self-doubt. For many of us, the confusion around this question is excruciating.

—ANDREW COHEN, American spiritual teacher

When it comes to sex and all its diversity, the one thing everyone has in common is to wonder, "Am I normal?" Most of us have no way of knowing how to compare ourselves to someone else. As teenagers and young adults there may be a fair amount of braggadocio among men, and talk about sexual hookups as conquests, but honest discussions between men about their sexual experiences is rare. I believe a man's sense of masculinity is fragile in large part because there is little knowledge of what is true about men and sex.

Sizing Things Up

Marvin was a very pleasant sixty-seven-year-old man who had undergone radiation treatment for prostate cancer ten years earlier. Since that time, his cancer had been in remission, but the radiation had caused his erections to worsen and then fail, and seven years ago he had opted for a penile implant. Marvin had an unusual demeanor. He spoke very slowly and deliberately. He had a bemused attitude toward life and a wisdom that was almost Talmudic.

When I saw him for a routine follow-up this past year, I asked, "How are things going with the implant? Are you having sex?"

"Doctor, you have just asked me two separate questions. Please allow me to answer each of them separately. I will begin with the second question. I am not having sex. My wife takes approximately 230 medications a day. She has no interest. By now, it is an old story. I suppose if I pleaded my case she might accommodate me. However, it is not enjoyable to have sex with a woman if she has no interest. I'm not delighted by my situation, but what can I do?

"For younger couples," Marvin continued, "if there is no sex maybe they're better off with someone else. But when a couple has been together as long as we have, there are other things that keep the relationship going besides sex. It would be nice to have that great feeling, that excitement, once in a while, but our relationship doesn't depend on those experiences anymore.

"Now, as to your second question, or rather your first, which I've elected to answer second, the implant itself is fine. I take it out for a spin now and again, to check and see if the equipment is functioning, and that my own internal organs still do what they were designed to do. It's a bit like a middle-aged divorced man driving a red convertible sports car with the top down. If there's no one in the street to watch him drive by, it is a reasonably good experience, but empty. I was hoping that the implant would bring my penis back to its original size. It's become smaller as I got older. But other than that, it works and I have no complaints."

This was the first time Marvin had ever commented on the size of his penis.

"Marvin," I explained, "the reason your penis isn't as large as when you were younger is that the radiation treatments cause scarring of the tissues. They become less elastic, so the erection can't expand the penis to the same size."

"It's all right, Doctor. I'm not really complaining. You know, I had always been annoyed that I was short, at five foot six. However, I had an uncle who was five foot five. He told me that he also used to be very annoyed that he was short until he went into the army. One day he's in battle, and the guy behind him, who was six feet tall, gets his head blown off. From that day forward, he told me, it didn't bother him that he was five foot five. We have to make peace with the way things are."

Men are funny about the size of their penises. They compare, when they can. In the shower at the gym where men see each other naked, you can see each man putting on a show of not being interested in checking out the penises of other men, yet still trying to catch a glimpse if they think they won't get caught doing it. It is a reckoning of sorts, trying to figure out where they stand with their own penis.

Thanks to my work I have probably seen as many penises as anyone else in the world, sometimes as many as fifty in a day. Not just glancing looks from afar but detailed looks under bright lights as part of an examination. And yet one evening in a restaurant bathroom, after a long day with patients, I caught myself glancing down at the guy at the adjacent urinal! I nearly burst out laughing at myself. If there is anyone alive who does *not* need to check out one more penis, it is me. It's a male reflex.

The male obsession with size is related to the belief that a larger penis makes a man more desirable, more powerful. In my experience, men are anxious about being seen naked if they believe their penis is small, but if they believe they have something large hiding in their underpants, they are very quick, sometimes comically so, to drop their trousers. Confidence is paramount when it comes to sex, and a man's assessment of his penis size has an outsized effect on that confidence.

A common problem for men is they think their penis is small even when it isn't. In studies where men are asked whether they believe their penis is smaller than average, average, or larger than average, as many as 75 percent respond that their penis is smaller than average. Since it is statistically impossible for 75 percent of men to be below average, this means that either men have a skewed ability to assess themselves, or they have a misguided notion of what an "average" penis looks like.

One day, a longtime patient of mine asked me if I would see his twenty-five-year-old son, Charlie. "He had an undescended testicle removed when he was a child, and he's very self-conscious about having only one testicle," the father said. Charlie had finished college, was a smart kid, but he still lived at home in their basement. He worked occasional shifts at a comic book store. Although he used to be fairly social, his father said he never went out anymore, not even with his old friends. And, his father added, Charlie did not date, despite being a "good-looking kid."

When Charlie came to see me in the office, I said, "Your father told me you were concerned about having just one testicle. Is that right?"

"That's part of it," he answered. "The thing I'm more worried about, though, is that my penis is too small."

"Why do you say that?"

"I just think it is. Can you make it bigger?"

On examination the left testicle was absent, but the right one was fine. And Charlie's penis wasn't small at all. Flaccid, it was 4.5 inches, slightly larger than average (which is, according to some studies, around 3.5 inches—but more on that later in this chapter). "Charlie," I began after he had dressed and was seated in front of me, "your examination is perfectly normal, apart from the fact that you're missing one testicle. You'd be surprised how many men have just one. They go on to live perfectly normal lives, and I expect you to as well. The testicles make two things—testosterone and sperm—and one good testicle is all a man needs for those."

Charlie was listening intently.

"As for your penis, you've got a *great* penis. Many men I see would love to have a penis as big as yours."

"That's hard to believe," he said. "I've seen guys in X-rated movies, and they all have penises that are way bigger than mine."

"Charlie, you can't compare yourself to the guys in porn movies. Most of those men are freaks of nature. They are selected for those movies exactly because they have an unusually large penis. It's certainly not because of their acting skills!" I joked. "Listen, no one compares well to those guys."

Charlie nodded. "I know," he said. "I go to the gym once in a while. You see other guys in the shower. I've never seen anyone as big as the guys in the movies. They really are freaks."

"Charlie, have you had sex?" I asked.

"Yes, a couple of times."

"I'm curious why you think your penis is small."

Charlie was quiet for a moment, then spoke up. "I've only had sex with two girls. The last one, we just had sex once. I barely knew her. She said something as she was leaving that sounded like she was making fun of my penis. That was, like, five years ago. I haven't had sex since then."

"Did you think your penis was small before that day?"

"No."

"Charlie, people say awful things. It doesn't mean they're true. I'm sorry that girl said something cruel to you, but you need to forget what she said. Listen, I see penises all day long, and I assure you that your penis is fine. In fact, it's above average in size."

Charlie didn't have much of a reaction to what I said. I invited him to visit me again in a couple of months, but he never came back. About a year later I saw Charlie's father for a routine appointment. When we were done, I asked about his son.

"Doctor, I don't know what you said to Charlie last year, but you're a magician. I meant to tell you about him. A few weeks after he saw you he found a good job, moved out of the house, and got his own apartment. He started going out again, and he's got a girlfriend now. It's been a complete transformation."

All Charlie needed was reassurance that his penis was all right.

Making the Most of What You Have

How long should a penis be? Practically speaking, an erect penis needs to be long enough to reach inside a woman's vagina. That may not sound like a very high bar to reach, but there are rare cases where even this is a problem.

Some men are born with a penis that is truly too small, called a micropenis, but this is extremely rare. It is defined by an erection that is less than two inches in length. Obesity can cause the penis to "hide" within the surrounding fat, but the penis itself is fine in those cases. A colleague presented data at a meeting that obese men gain an average of one inch of visible penis for every thirty-five pounds they lose. Now there's a good reason to diet! A more serious problem is when there's been a trauma or cancer that requires surgery to remove a portion of the penis. For the surgeon, the rule of thumb is to try to leave a minimum of two inches so that the penis can be "functional." This length allows the man to direct his stream when he urinates, and to reach the vagina and move in and out a bit during sex.

Hal was thirty-six when he first came to see me. He was a muscular, exceedingly polite construction worker, "all man," one would think, with a plaid lumberjack shirt with ragged sleeves cut short showing off huge biceps. Hal had been born with a devastating condition called exstrophy (pronounced "ex-trophy," with the emphasis on the first syllable, as in "ecstasy"). Infants born with exstrophy have a developmental problem in which the abdominal muscles don't develop properly, and the pubic bones are wide apart instead of having fused in the midline as they normally do. The most obvious and dramatic abnormality, however, is that the bladder sits open on the front of the abdomen, external to the body. These babies undergo surgery to close their bladders and create space for them inside the pelvis. In some cases, however, the bladders are only rudimentary, and the best choice is to remove it entirely and create an alternative way for the urine to come out. In Hal's infancy, his bladder was removed, and the ureters, the tubes that bring urine down from the kidneys, were rerouted to drain into his colon. This meant that every time Hal had a bowel movement, he urinated. And vice versa.

Exstrophy is particularly hard on males once they grow up, because they often have an additional problem with a deformed and unusually small penis. Since the two corpora cavernosa are anchored to the underside of the pubic bone, and because the two halves of the pubic bones are so far apart in these cases, much of the length of the corpora cavernosa is spent just reaching to the midline to join the other side. Length that would normally go to create the visible shaft of the penis is hidden inside and under the separated pubic bones.

Hal's penis was very short, at about two inches, and he had extensive scar tissue along the upper portion that caused the penis to curve severely upward when it became erect . The tip of Hal's erect penis tickled the lower part of his abdomen, like a miniature boomerang. Between the curve and the short penis, there was no way Hal could have intercourse.

Hal came to see me once a year for three years to discuss what could be done surgically to have a penis that would allow him to penetrate a vagina. After his third visit and a lot of hand-wringing, he decided to do it.

I wanted to accomplish two things with the surgery: One was to free up the two corpora cavernosa from the scar tissue that held them back and also to free them from the underside of each half of the pubic bones. This would give Hal more length. The second was to tighten up the underside of the corpora cavernosa so that the penis would be straighter. At the end of the procedure Hal had just over three inches, and his erection pointed outward from his body for the first time in his life.

"Doctor, my erection is so much better," Hal said, when I saw him for a follow-up one month after surgery. "But it still seems awfully short. Do you think I've got enough to be able to have sex?"

"Sure," I replied. "Is there someone you're planning on trying it out with?"

"Not really."

"Well, you've healed up nicely. You've got the green light from me to go ahead and have sex."

Hal returned three months later for another follow-up. All was going well, but he still hadn't had sex.

I didn't see Hal again for about two years. He was now forty-one. He seemed happy and less revved up than I'd seen him before. Interestingly, he wasn't wearing anything that showed off his muscles anymore.

"Have you had sex yet?" I asked, though I expected the same answer I'd heard in his last two visits. Even when a man goes through a major event, such as surgery, to fix something like this, the physical part is only a piece of the action. Socially, mentally, it can be difficult to switch gears, to go from feeling like a "freak," as Hal had put it in an early conversation with me, to feeling comfortable enough to put himself out there with a woman.

"I have!" answered Hal enthusiastically. He seemed pleased with himself.

"Great," I said. "How did it go?"

"Doctor, I hope there's no ten-thousand-mile limit on the work you did, because the truth is I've been wearing my penis out. First, I took a chance with this girl I knew. I was nervous that she'd laugh at me because my dick was too short, but it worked out great. It was amazing to finally be able to have sex after all these years. We did it a couple of times. Then I saw another girl for a while. Right now I'm dating a woman I really like. We have sex four, maybe five times a week! I know I don't have the longest dick in the world, but it seems to do the trick. I guess there's something to that old line, 'It's not the meat, it's the motion.'"

"When did you start having sex?" I asked.

"It was soon after my last visit with you, about two years ago. I was thirty-nine years old. Can you believe it? There I was, a thirty-nine-year-old man having sex for the first time. I'm not complaining; I was convinced it would never happen in my lifetime."

"Did you see the movie *The 40-Year-Old Virgin*?" I asked.

"I did! I laughed about that one a lot. I snuck in there just before he did!"

The Lengths Men Go To

Man's obsession with penis size is nothing new. As an adolescent on family vacation at the ruins of Pompeii, I remember my father paying the tour guide an extra fee to look at a special fresco behind a curtain. My mother and sister were not invited. Painted on the wall was the picture of a nobleman (some accounts say the character is Priapus, the Greek god of fertility) with an enormous erect penis, the length and girth larger than a man's leg, placed on an ancient scale, with sacks of gold balanced on the other side. I rediscovered that image on the Internet and have occasionally used it in lectures, with the quip that men have always viewed a large penis as worth its weight in gold.

The male preoccupation with penis size causes some men to pursue advertised treatments to help them enlarge their penis. Dustin was a thirty-three-year-old married man who bought a traction device online and used it for several months in the hope that it would make his penis longer. He came to see me because he was experiencing penile numbness, chronic discomfort, and a change in urination. The traction device attaches behind the head of the penis and the other end pushes against the pubic bone. Spacers are used to adjust the length, and the device then stretches the penis away from the body. The sales pitch is that the traction device will stretch the penis over time as much as two to three inches, which would be incredible if it were true. A minor drawback is that the man needs to wear the traction device for a minimum of four hours daily. That means putting it on as soon as one returns home from work. Or wearing the device under one's pants at work. That's dedication.

If it weren't a real product, the traction device would sound like a joke. Imagine a man's genitals stretched for hours at a time with a deviously engineered device that resembles the medieval torture mechanism the rack? Can you imagine if word got out that a captured al-Qaeda terrorist was forced to wear one of these? There would be protest marches in the street at this violation of the Geneva Conventions. Yet men do this voluntarily in the never-ending search for greater virility in the form of a longer penis.

There is no shortage of modern-day con men willing to take advantage of this obsession with penis size. Supplements and herbal concoctions are sold in stores and online with promises to increase a man's size. "Be the man you've always wanted to be," they say. Then there are the manipulation techniques that provide a more "organic" version of the penile rack. The most popular of these at the moment is called jelqing. Jelqing consists of massaging the penis outward while semierect to "push" more blood into the glans, thereby (according to jelqing proponents) causing the penis to expand. This makes no medical sense at all, but a brief Internet search leads to dozens of videos and instructional guides. One nineteen-year-old man, Louie, came to see me after a few episodes of jelqing, afraid that he had injured himself by being too enthusiastic in his technique.

Then there are the pumps. These are similar to the vacuum erection devices used to treat ED. A plastic cylinder is placed over the penis and air is pumped out of the cylinder, causing blood to move into the penis and creating an artificial erection. The famed comedic movie ladies' man Austin Powers used a Swedish penis pump to keep himself in tiptop shape. And back in the reality-based world, an Oklahoma judge, Donald Thompson, was convicted of indecency due to his habit of using a penis pump behind the bench while presiding over criminal cases.

It's easy enough to understand why a man might want to have a larger penis. The question is what impels him to actually do something about it when the solutions are so obviously fantasy-based. For some men, it is a feeling of masculine inadequacy. Dustin, aka Mr. Traction Device, couldn't answer my question directly when I asked why he had been using this device. However, it turned out that his wife had cheated on him. Louie, aka Mr. Jelqing, explained that he tried the technique because he "thought it would be cool to have a bigger penis." At nineteen, his sexual experience was limited to two very brief "hookups," none within the last year. He thought it was possible that a larger penis might make him more appealing to women. Ironically, Louie's penis was already quite generous in size.

It is common for men to assume that difficulties in a relationship stem directly from their performance in bed. Some men may believe that by taking Viagra or enlarging their penis they can win back the hearts of their partner, even though nonsexual issues (e.g., alcoholism, abusiveness, lack of affection) are more likely causes for a partner to stray sexually or to break off a relationship.

Men may believe it would be great to have a huge penis, but it's not necessarily so. Take Peter, for example, a fifty-two-year-old Web site developer in whom I placed a penile implant for ED. He was a serious, thoughtful man. And he had one of the largest penises I've seen: a full eight inches erect. At surgery he required the longest implant available, and I had to add several spacers to allow the implant to fit properly. At a follow-up visit I asked whether he was aware he was unusually large.

"Yes," he said. "My wife and I go to a nude beach every summer, and I've never seen anyone with a longer penis than me. I've known since middle school that I was bigger than most guys. The other boys made a lot of comments about my penis."

"Did that make you proud? Make you feel like you had some kind of male advantage over them?" I asked.

"Not at all," Peter answered quietly. "I was terribly embarrassed by it. The boys would say, 'If you ever have sex with a girl, you're going to come out the other side.' I felt like a freak."

"What about when you were older and more experienced? Was your penis a source of pride then?"

"No. I was as awkward with girls as anyone else. I don't understand the obsession with penis size."

I've always been impressed by the number of men I've seen with serious medical challenges who are accompanied by attractive women. In some of these cases the men are unable to function sexually, yet their partners are devoted to them. One lesson women have been trying to tell men for a long time is, "It's not about the penis; it's about the man the penis is attached to."

As obvious as this message may sound, it may not get through to a young man just learning the complex rules of sexual engagement. And when there has been a blow to a man's ego, for example, when a man finds a girlfriend has cheated or simply moved on to another man, it is commonplace for the man to blame it on his penis or his inadequacies as a lover. No wonder, then, that men frequently succumb to the seductive charms of the Sirens of the Internet, promising incredible virility, instant sex appeal, and eternal happiness ($49.99/month, credit card required).

Okay, But How Do I Stack Up?

So, what is a normal penis size? In a study performed at the University of California in San Francisco, doctors measured penis size in eighty volunteers. They measured penises flaccid (soft), as soon as the subjects dropped their trousers, and they measured them erect. The erections were achieved pharmacologically, by penile injection of the same medications used to treat ED. The average flaccid length, measured from the point where the skin of the penis meets the body to the tip of the penis, averaged 8.9 centimeters, or 3.5 inches, with a range of 2 to 6 inches. Erect penises averaged 12.9 centimeters, or just over 5 inches. The shortest penis in this group of men was 3 inches, and the longest was 7.6 inches. The average increase in length from flaccid to erect was 4.0 centimeters, or a bit more than 1.5 inches. Some men had a substantial increase in length, as much as 3.5 inches, whereas others had almost none.

Men with smaller penises had on average the same amount of growth with erections as men with larger penises, contrary to lore that smaller penises lengthen more. However, there is some truth to the concept if one considers proportional growth. For example, a man with a 3-inch penis when flaccid who gains the average amount of 1.5 inches will have increased his length by 50 percent, whereas a man with a flaccid length of 6 inches who gains the same 1.5 inches will have added only 25 percent to his flaccid length. So perhaps it is still all right to say that "some men are grow-ers, and some men are show-ers." And of course, all men experience shrinkage when cold or nervous, which would make their subsequent erection when aroused appear to be even more substantial.

Can I Make It Last All Night, Every Night?

Gary was a fifty-six-year-old sales director who wanted to discuss his symptoms of low testosterone with me. His wife of thirty-four years, Anna, accompanied him. She was one year younger than he was. Gary told me that his energy was way down, and he felt constantly fatigued. "Recently, I've taken to sleeping a minimum of nine hours a day just to be able to make it through the day," he said. "And my sex drive is way down. My erections aren't that great either. We only have sex now about once a week."

"When did you notice a change in your sex drive?" I asked.

"I'd say about nine months ago," Gary replied.

Anna looked at Gary, then at me. "Doctor, may I say something?" she said. "Gary has *always* had a low sex drive. On our honeymoon, if you can believe it, he sent me home with a couple of his coworkers! That's not normal!"

"I don't understand," I said to Anna. "What were coworkers doing on your honeymoon?"

"We were at a resort on a lake about two hours from where we lived. A couple of guys from Gary's work were traveling nearby, so he arranged for them to stop by for dinner, and then they drove me back home to stay with my folks."

"In my defense," said Gary, "it wasn't a traditional honeymoon. It was more of a working trip that we took right after we got married. We stayed at a nice resort near where I had to do some work with clients. We would have sex in the morning before I left for the field, again when I came back for lunch, and then again when I came back at the end of the day. Anna would come to bed at the end of the night as late as midnight, and even though I had to go to work in the morning, we would do it again. After two or three days of that, I thought it was perfectly reasonable to send her home for a few days to stay with her family so I could get some rest!"

This topic was a bit delicate. I explained that one of the challenges within a relationship arises when one person enjoys sex on a more frequent schedule than the other. Until recently it was assumed that it was always the man who wanted sex more than the woman, but in my practice I've seen plenty of couples in which the woman is the driver. It can be a problem for both partners. One feels that he or she is being deprived, and the other feels put upon.

I told Gary and Anna about a scene in the movie *Annie Hall* (1977), where the Woody Allen character and his girlfriend, played by Diane Keaton, are both seeing their respective psychiatrists at the same time. Allen laments, "We never have sex," to his therapist, while Keaton complains, "We're constantly having sex," to her therapist. Both shrinks ask, "How often do you have sex?" And both Allen and Keaton answer, "Three times a week."

Neither Gary nor Anna betrayed any emotion as I told this story. Maybe they didn't find the story as amusing as I did.

Gary's blood tests later showed low levels of testosterone, and I treated him. I was curious whether the treatments would affect his libido. After a few months, Gary and Anna came back to see me.

"I feel better in general, I'd say," reported Gary. "Energy, mood. I'm sleeping better too and don't need to sleep as long to feel rested."

"What about sex?" I asked.

"Oh that!" said Gary, with a chuckle. "Yup, that's better too. I'd forgotten that was the original reason I came to see you."

"In what way is it better?"

"All of it, I would say. Desire, drive, libido—whatever you want to call it. Erections are easier to get and easier to maintain too. I'd say we're doing okay in that department, wouldn't you?" he asked, turning to Anna, seated beside him.

"He's better," Anna responded, addressing herself to me. "I'm not going to say it's where I think it should be, but we're back to having sex about as often as we used to a couple of years ago."

"How often is that?" I asked.

"Three times a week," they both answered in unison.

There's no right answer to the question "How often should I be having sex?" There is so much variation in what feels right from person to person.

The frequency with which we have sex is influenced by a number of factors. Younger men tend to have sex more than older men, but not by as much as one would think. A recent online survey of 522 men between the ages of twenty-one and fifty-nine published in *Esquire* magazine reported that 32 percent of respondents claimed to have sex one to three times per week, and another 33 percent had it less than once a week. And in a study of men and women older than fifty-seven years published in the *New England Journal of Medicine*, of those who were partnered and sexually active, roughly 60 percent of the men reported having sex at least two to three times per month. The figures were similar for women. In a study of sexual patterns in 27,500 men and women ages forty to eighty years from twenty-nine countries, Alfred Nicolosi and his colleagues reported that 44 percent of men and 38 percent of women engaged in intercourse more than once a week. A bigger issue as we age is that a substantial number of men and women stop having sex altogether. In men the most common reason is erectile dysfunction. In women the most common reason given is lack of sexual interest, which becomes much more prevalent after menopause.

Sex is far more frequent when a relationship is new than when it is three to five years old. The big surprise for many readers is that men with long-term partners, married or not, have more sex than single men. In one survey, single men were twice as likely as married men to go one to three months without sex. The married man (or woman) may complain that he (or she) doesn't get *enough* sex, but in the vast majority of cases there is already an existing sexual relationship in which sex does occur with some frequency. In contrast, the single man who wants to have sex has to first find a partner.

Zachary is an example of a married man who had stopped having sex. When he came into my office for a routine visit, he was ninety-one, still mentally sharp, and still married to his first wife, who was eighty-six. He was dressed in jogging pants and sported a two- to three-day-old beard.

"I haven't had sex in twenty years," he told me.

"What about an orgasm? Can you still come?"

"No. I haven't had one of those in about fifteen years."

"Do you miss it?"

"Sure, but I'm not twenty-one anymore. Let me tell you something. When I was seventeen I used to go get my hair cut at the barber shop by this Italian guy. He was probably about twenty-one. One day he tells me about his wedding night. He had sex seven times that night, he says. You know, I still have dreams of not satisfying a woman sexually, and I think it came from listening to that barber. It made a big impression on me. I hadn't even had sex yet, but I held that guy's experience up as a standard. When I was in my twenties I could usually do it twice. Maybe once in my life I did it three times."

He looked pensive for a minute and then said, "You know sometimes you hear guys talk about 'screwing their brains out'? I never screwed my brains out. All in all, though, I think I did okay by my wife. She seemed satisfied."

"Could your wife have an orgasm?"

"Oh, yeah. Most of the time. Not always."

"I still look at girls," he continued. "That's never stopped. And then I tell myself, 'Who am I kidding?' It's like a dog chasing a car. What's he going to do with it when he catches it? Anyway, no more sex for me. I still play tennis, though. I'm not great, but guys at the club still ask me to play. I only play doubles. Life is strange. Nearly everyone I know has died, and here I am playing tennis. Go figure."

Zachary's story is poignant in many ways. It's fascinating to me that even at ninety-one he was still bothered by an experience that happened to him at seventeen, in which his idea of what was normal was created by a slightly older man who had had an evening of incredible sex that Zachary could never replicate. As a result, he saw himself as sexually deficient his entire life, despite having what sounded like a thoroughly satisfactory, even enviable, sexual relationship with his wife over several decades.

The need to constantly measure oneself against some impossibly high standard of masculinity leaves too many men feeling deficient. Men care enormously about their sexual proficiency, yet in the absence of real information it is easy for them to feel that they don't quite match up.

The number of orgasms a man can have in one night or within twenty-four hours is highly variable. Men require a certain amount of time to reload and recharge. When they are young, it can be a few minutes. In their thirties and forties, it usually takes much longer, often hours, and some completely healthy young men find it impossible to have more than one orgasm until the next day. In the older years, it may take up to a week to recharge.

Relationships Without Sex

Some couples who are decades younger than Zachary and his wife don't have sex at all. Scott was fifty-two and had been on testosterone for years under my care. His girlfriend of ten years, Jill, was forty-four. When I asked Scott whether he was having sex these days, he told me no.

"Why not?" I asked.

"Jill is kinda religious," he answered.

"That's a reason to not have sex?"

"I don't know. I think she's bothered by the fact that I never married her, after all these years."

"Is she angry about it?"

"*I* think so. She doesn't say that, though, and she doesn't really show it."

"Are you okay with not having sex?"

"It's all right. It's just the way it is. Jill is a great person. Salt of the earth. Everyone likes her. I don't think it's right that we don't have sex. Every time I've thought of moving on, though, it was me who came back to her. We stay together on the weekends and live in our own places during the week. Before we got together she raised her children on her own as a single mother. She had a female roommate when I met her. Even when we did have sex at the beginning, it was only once or twice a week."

"Did you want to have sex more then?"

"Sure! Jill was never that interested, though. It seemed like she was doing it mainly for me."

I never met Jill, so I can't say why she was reluctant to have sex with Scott. Maybe Jill just didn't enjoy sex. Maybe her religious training soured her on sex or made her feel uncomfortable with it outside of a marriage, as Scott had suggested initially. Maybe she had withheld sex from Scott out of anger. Perhaps she had been sexually abused as a child. Maybe she was gay. There could be any number of reasons.

What is important to note, though, is that Scott's situation is not particularly unusual. There are many couples who don't have sex or have sex only rarely. For every Anna, with a lifelong high-frequency desire, there are other women who don't care for sex with their partner. So when men ask me, "How often should I be having sex?" there is no ready answer. Statistics show that the average married couple has sex approximately once per week, with rates higher among younger couples and more recent marriages, and declining with age and years of marriage.

What If I Don't Do It at All?

Not everyone wants to have sex. Simon was a seventy-five-year-old psychiatrist who described himself as a lifelong bachelor, a term one doesn't hear much nowadays. Simon was a nice-looking, neatly dressed older man, with a full head of longish, white hair, a touch of pomade holding it back. He swam five days a week and appeared quite fit. I asked Simon what he meant by *lifelong bachelor*.

"Well, I guess it means that I've always been on my own. Never married."

"Did you have partners in the past? Relationships?"

"I dated a bit in college but didn't have sex. In the 1980s I had sex with one woman, three times. And that's been it."

"What's it been like to be alone all these years?"

"I'm used to it. It's not so bad really. Better than the alternative."

"What do you mean by that?"

"I have what would now be called social anxiety disorder. I'm self-diagnosed, of course. For me, being alone is far preferable to the anxiety I would have experienced with women. Some colleagues probably think I've remained unmarried because I'm secretly gay, but I assure you I'm not. My fantasies are all about women."

"What about sex? Do you miss that?"

"Not really. I didn't enjoy it much the few times I did have it. There was too much pressure for me trying to satisfy the woman while trying to satisfy myself. I found all of it uncomfortable: the courting, the lead-up to becoming intimate, the conversation, or nonconversation, that led us finally to bed. The undressing. What to say to her as she was becoming naked, what she might think of me as I undressed. It was too much. No, I can't say I've missed it at all. So I have sex by myself. Me and my hand, as it were."

We moved on to other aspects of Simon's medical status, and during a review of his medications, I noticed he was taking finasteride, frequently prescribed in middle-aged and older men to help with frequent urination due to an enlarged prostate. I asked Simon if finasteride had been helpful for his urination.

"Finasteride?" he asked. "I don't take that for my prostate. I take it for my hair, to prevent hair loss."

"Really?" I said in surprise. "I'm surprised to hear that given what you've just told me."

"Perhaps it's egotistic of me," Simon replied, "but I do still like it when I get a compliment. If a woman tells me I look good, it makes my day."

Even small, daily-life interactions with women can be enormously important to men, even if there is nothing overtly sexual about it. One additional point to take away from Simon's touching story is that everyone enjoys a compliment. If I were restricted to one single tip to help men and women in their intimate relationships it is this: find something nice to say to your partner every day. Compliments can be large or small, but details make the appreciation more believable, for example, "I like those shoes" or "That dress is a great color for you." Of course, there's never anything wrong with saying, "You look handsome tonight" or "You're so beautiful."

12. NO BALLS AT ALL

Wealth is nothing, position is nothing, fame is nothing, manhood is everything.

—ORISON SWETT MARDEN, American physician and philosopher, 1850–1924

After All These Years

When I was a young surgeon on the staff of my hospital I read that a new physician had joined the surgical staff. By his distinctive name—let's call him Chas—I recognized him as the boy who had grown up across the street from me. We were the same age, and we had competed against each other in an endless variety of neighborhood games after school and on weekends. He had always acted superior, and I had never liked him very much. One day when we were about eleven, things came to a head: He claimed to have won a race that I had clearly won. I told him I had won. He pushed me, and I pushed him back. We wrestled, and I pinned him to the ground. As I did, he spit in my face and then scurried away as I wiped his disgusting saliva from my cheek. He avoided me after that episode. Twenty-four years later, here we were at the same hospital, as colleagues.

As soon as I saw his name I instantly remembered our boy-hood unpleasantness. Then I scolded myself for my reaction, thinking that it was ridiculous to hold any negative feelings toward someone who was a child at the time, and I determined to be friendly. I sent Chas an e-mail welcoming him to the institution, and he wrote back with a polite thank-you.

A short while later I ran into Chas in the radiology depart-ment, at the window where physicians requested X-rays on their patients. He looked more or less as I would have expected, about the same height as me, but a bit stockier. He was a serious man, and I thought I detected the same whiff of superiority he'd had as a youngster, but I dismissed it as my own prejudice against him. I asked him about his work, and he told me he specialized in the new field of brain surgery for seizure disorders. He asked me about mine, and I told him I specialized in treating men with reproductive and sexual issues.

"Do you have any kids?" Chas asked.

"Not yet," I said.

"That's not much of a recommendation for you, is it?" He smirked. "I've got three." He then abruptly turned his back to me and walked away, apparently pleased with his zinger. After all these years, he was still an asshole.

I would like to be able to say that Chas's words didn't bother me. They did, though. I knew that I didn't need to have children of my own to be an infertility specialist, just as one doesn't need to have cancer to be a good oncologist. Nonetheless, the remark stung, and I played that brief interaction over and over in my head for a long time. I know Chas's put-down had nothing to do with my professional abilities—what could he have known about them? Rather, it was an attack on my manhood. Manhood as defined by fathering children. Ultimately, by having balls. This is what we men do to each other. We compete and we tease each other; we con-stantly evaluate ourselves against other men, trying to figure out our position on the totem pole. Because no matter how successful we are, in whatever realm, all men are vulnerable when it comes to their manhood.

When we think about what makes a man a man, the first thing that pops into mind is the penis. However, biologically, and perhaps socially too, it is the testicles that are most associated with masculinity. We talk about men having "balls" as a mark of courage. The same is true for other cultures, other languages; the Spanish word *cojones*, for example. Any farmer, rancher, or veterinarian knows, too, that male animals behave differently with and without testicles.

The importance of the testicles to men is underscored by the words *testify* and *testimony*, which are derived from *testis*. There is evidence going back to the Greeks, Romans, and even the biblical Israelites that placing one's hand upon one's testicles was a way of assuring a court that one was telling the truth. A passage from Genesis in the King James translation of the Bible, reads, "And Abraham said unto his eldest servant of his house, that ruled over all that he had, 'Put, I pray thee, thy hand under my thigh.'" This passage suggests that a variation was to have someone else put their hand down there, making one a bit, shall we say, vulnerable? One description of this custom suggested that allowing others to place their hands upon one's testicles was proof that one was a man, especially a virile man. Since castration was performed as a punishment for certain crimes, the presence of testicles helped to demonstrate a level of trustworthiness.

"I'll Take Two Large Balls, Please"

Richard was what one would call a "high energy" type. He was the forty-six-year-old owner of several fast-food franchises, and when he sat in the exam room I could almost feel him vibrate. Funny and engaging, he was one of those guys who couldn't keep still. He was very fit and tall, with a set of very white teeth that gleamed whenever he cracked one of his frequent jokes.

This was Richard's third annual visit with me. Every year we discussed the same thing, but this time he brought his wife with him. "I'm ready for the operation now," he said to me. "That's why I brought MaryAnne with me. We both have questions we'd like to discuss with you."

MaryAnne was an attractive, warmhearted woman. She worked as a nurse in the operating room at a local hospital and had come to the appointment wearing her surgical scrubs. Mary-Anne didn't quite have Richard's energy level—not many people could—but she had a lot of spirit herself, and kept up with him.

When he was eighteen, Richard's right testicle was removed when his doctors discovered cancer. At thirty-seven, he developed a lump in the left testicle; it too was cancerous, and the doctors removed it. Fortunately, the cancer hadn't spread. Once the second testicle was removed, Richard's body was unable to make any testosterone, and his physician prescribed weekly testosterone injections to allow him to function normally—sexually and otherwise.

"Before that second operation," Richard said, "I asked if they could just take out the part of my nut with the cancer and leave me something there in my sac, so I wouldn't be left with absolutely nothing. The doctors said 'no,' it wasn't worth taking the chance of leaving any cancer behind. They didn't have any choice, they said. They needed to be sure. I knew that. I was the one who found the lump. I didn't want to die. 'Okay, take it out,' I said to the doctors. They did the operation. Here I am, almost ten years later, and everything is all right except for one thing."

"What's that?" I asked.

"Doc!" he exclaimed, "I've got no balls! No balls at all! How can a guy feel good about himself without balls? I put my hand down my pants ten, twenty times a day. It's not right for a guy to have nothing there."

MaryAnne pitched in. "It's true, Doctor," she said. "He is always feeling down there. At home, his hands are always in his pants."

Richard interjected, "Of course, I'm not saying I wasn't doing that before, too."

MaryAnne continued, "I think Richard has magical thoughts, hoping that one day he'll feel down there and find something again."

"Yeah," he added. "Like, 'Hey honey! Look what I found!'"

They both laughed. They were like a comedy duo.

"Doc, every year I talk to you about those artificial balls. Testicular implants. I'm ready now. The other doc offered to put them in when he was going to take out the second testicle, but I hated the idea of something artificial like that going in my body. MaryAnne and I are so careful about what we eat. Everything is organic. If we don't put anything artificial in our bodies normally, why would I want a piece of plastic put into me with an operation? 'No way,' I told him. Now, though, I'm ready to do it."

"What has changed for you?" I asked.

"Not having any balls affects me mentally. I don't feel right," he told me. "I go to the gym every day, but I don't shower there. I go home. No way I'm going to let those guys I work out with know I don't have any balls."

"So you want the implants so you'll look better in the shower with other guys?" I asked.

"No, no," Richard answered animatedly. "This is for me. I don't really care what those guys think. They're all lunkheads anyway."

"I thought they were your friends," MaryAnne teased him.

"They are. They *are* my friends. They're also lunkheads," Richard replied. "I was just using that as an example. Listen, my life is going great. I've got the best wife ever, we have a blast together, the kids are fine. Work is good. The only thing that's wrong in my life is that I don't feel good about myself. I don't know how to describe it other than saying that my empty nut-sack makes me feel like I'm not a complete man. "

"Doctor, just so you know, I've told Richard I'm against this," MaryAnne said. "I've told him he's the best man I could ever have hoped to meet. He's fought cancer twice and beat it both times. He adopted my two kids from a previous relationship. That's what a real man does—he steps up, takes life as it is, and deals with it. I think he's nuts to do this."

"Nuts!" echoed Richard. "That's a good one. You think I'm nuts, but I don't have any nuts."

MaryAnne elbowed him in the side good-naturedly. "Anyway," she said, turning for a moment toward Richard with a look that suggested he shouldn't interrupt her anymore, "I've told Richard that he doesn't need to do this. Certainly not for me. He's every bit a man. The testosterone lets him be a regular guy. I give him the shots every week. Our sex life is fine."

"C'mon, honey!" Richard interjected yet again. "We're here with the doctor, and all you can say about our sex life is that it's *fine*? He turned toward me and in a slower, more deliberate voice said to me, with mock assurance, "Doctor, let me assure you, our sex life is better than 'fine.' It's great!"

"As I was saying," MaryAnne continued, "Richard is fine, and I've told him I don't see the need for him to have an operation with all its risks."

"What *are* the risks?" Richard asked.

"As MaryAnne knows from working in the hospital, there are risks to any operation, including bleeding, infection, pain."

"Will they look natural?" asked Richard.

"They usually look very good," I answered.

"What's it made out of?" Richard wanted to know.

"There are two types of implants," I explained. "The one I prefer is made out of silicone gel. It mimics the feel of a real testicle. The other is saline. It's a hollow oval that is filled with salt water."

"Aren't there problems with silicone implants?" asked Richard.

"Not really," I answered. "Years ago there was a big hullabaloo about silicone breast implants in women, and they were taken off the market for a while. Studies have shown that it wasn't a real problem, though, so they're back on the market again. And there had never been any problems in men with silicone implants anyway."

"They started doing silicone breast implants again at my hospital about five years ago," said MaryAnne. "The surgeons say they're just as safe and give a more natural result."

I brought out samples of both kinds of implants.

"This one is good!" said Richard admiringly as he held the silicone implant. It looked and felt like a shelled hard-boiled egg. "It feels real. Although how would I know, since I don't have any to compare to," he noted wryly. "The other one, the saline one, feels like a miniature bag of water."

"Do these come in different sizes?" asked MaryAnne.

Richard stopped playing and paid attention.

"Yes, they do," I replied. "Basically, they come in small, medium, and large sizes."

"I'll take two large balls, please," requested Richard. "Make those 'to go.'"

"I'll tell you what," I said. "If you decide to go forward with this, I'll give you the largest ones that will look natural in your scrotum. Deal?"

"Deal!" agreed Richard.

Richard had the surgery. Under general anesthesia I made an incision on his right side, a little higher than the top of the scrotum. I then created a path into the lowest part of the scrotum by inserting one and then two fingers, and spreading them apart. I rinsed out this newly created scrotal space with antibiotic solution.

Next I took a clamp and, with the jaws closed, pushed up on the lowest part of the scrotum, inverting it, and bringing it up into the wound. With the inside of the scrotum facing me, I placed a stitch into the muscular scrotal lining and then took a stitch into a patch on the implant specially designed for this. I tied down the suture, affixing the lower part of the artificial testicle to the lowest part of the sac, leaving a little room so that the testicle would have a small amount of freedom to move within the scrotum once it was in place. By pulling down gently on the scrotal skin from below and pushing gently from above, I popped the implant through the small skin incision and gave it a new home within the right side of the scrotum. It was the large size, and it fit nicely. I sutured the incision closed and then repeated the same maneuver on the other side.

"Wow," said the scrub nurse. "Those implants look so natural." It was a nice result, and I hoped Richard would be happy with it.

Richard and MaryAnne came back to see me a month after surgery. To show me how he had healed up, Richard pulled off his T-shirt and dropped his trousers, showing off his muscular physique and newly dangling implants. "Doc, I've got balls again!"

"Doctor," said MaryAnne, "I know it's only a month, but I've got to tell you, I already see a big change in Richard."

"What have you noticed?" I asked.

"He's calmer. He seems more at ease with himself. I hadn't expected this. Remember I told you I didn't think he needed the operation? If I'd known he'd be this way, I would have encouraged him to do it sooner. Richard jokes around so much that it's hard to know what's really going on inside his head, but I don't think I ever appreciated just how much it bothered him. He told you he wouldn't undress at the gym. The truth is, he wouldn't undress in front of me! He was okay with sex, but we used to do it in the dark. Or he got into bed before me. Now he walks around naked in front of me like it's no big deal. I think he *likes* to let me see him undressed now."

"I do, honey! Want me to show you again?" Richard said, turning toward her and pretending to unbutton his pants again.

"Did you know," continued MaryAnne to me, "when Richard went in to have his second testicle removed he told his family and the people at work that he had lymphoma? He didn't want them to know he had cancer of the testicle. And he hated anything that looked like balls."

"That's true, Doctor," said Richard. "One day we're driving along, and the truck in front of us has two big brass balls dangling from its rear. I'm going, 'Why is it me that gets stuck behind this goddamn truck with brass balls dangling?' Why couldn't he just have dice like everyone else?

"Doctor, can I tell you something weird? I know it doesn't make any sense, but the truth is that I felt *guilty* about not having balls. I believed deep down that I must have done something really bad in my life for this to happen. I'm better now. I know these fake balls aren't really mine, but they feel like they are. Makes me feel whole."

"What I Would Give for a Weekend With . . ."

She was beautiful. Elegant, regal, graceful. And he? He was in serious pain. Patrick was forty-two, and for weeks he had been planning a weekend getaway with the woman of his dreams, Celeste. He was an engineer, originally from Nigeria, and she was a thirty-four-year-old "haute" Haitian, a daughter of privilege, yet without any airs about her. Educated at Wellesley College, with a masters in education from Harvard, she was no dummy either. They had met, dated, and Patrick was so taken with Celeste that he would have done anything for her. Maybe he did.

Patrick had wanted the weekend in Montreal to be their first real romantic moment. He had made reservations at a gorgeous stone hotel in the Old City looking out over the St. Lawrence River, dinner at Les Halles, and an evening at a jazz bar known only to the cognoscenti for attracting the best in upcoming talent.

The pain in Patrick's right testicle began a few hours into the car ride. It started as a dull ache and grew in intensity, so that by the time they crossed the border, Patrick went to a convenience store to buy the souped-up Canadian version of over-the-counter pain killers called 222s. Codeine and acetaminophen, no prescription needed. There was no way Patrick was going to let this pain get in the way of his once-in-a-lifetime romantic getaway, even if his right testicle was swelling up badly. This was the woman, this was the moment.

It wasn't as if he didn't know what was going on. Patrick had experienced something very similar once before, about fifteen years earlier, on the left side. It had been the same kind of pain, the same sick feeling in the stomach, and the same swelling in the scrotum. Then, he ignored it until it went away, but afterward, his left testicle had shrunk to the size of a tiny bean. The pain and swelling had been caused by something called testicular torsion. It was a twist of the testicle on its own blood supply, leaving it necrotic. Dead. Now it was happening to the other side.

Patrick had toughed it out over the weekend despite the severe pain and swelling of his scrotum. By the time I saw him in the office, Celeste by his side, it had been about seventy-two hours since his symptoms began, and it was unlikely that I could save the testicles. It's unusual for a man to suffer long with that kind of pain. Usually, they show up in the emergency room right away, during that six- to eight-hour window of opportunity a doctor has in order to save the testicle. It needs to be untwisted, allowing return of blood to the testicle, and salvaging it.

When I examined Patrick, the scrotum was hugely swollen, to the size of a grapefruit. On the right side the skin was discolored, with red and purple areas. The testicle itself was also very swollen. It was a little tender, but not as much as I would have expected from how angry the scrotum looked. "It doesn't hurt as much as it did a couple of days ago," volunteered Patrick. An ultrasound confirmed there was no blood flow to the testicle.

"Patrick, you've had a torsion of your right testicle," I told him. "I wish you'd gone to get help in an emergency room when it first started because your testicle could have been saved with early treatment. Now, the damage has been done, and there's not much I can do. Your choice now is to go home with a prescription for pain medicine and rest, and over the next week or so the pain and swelling will improve. Or I can operate and remove the dead testicle. The advantage of an operation is usually a quicker recovery once the dead tissue is out of the body."

"Doctor, if you remove the testicle, will I still be able to have children?"

"I'm afraid not, Patrick. This was your last good testicle. The other one is too small to make sperm, and this one isn't working anymore. There's no way to make sperm without one good testicle."

"But Celeste won't marry me unless I can give her kids!" Patrick said in a loud whisper, not wanting Celeste to hear from outside the exam room.

"I'm sorry," I said. "I don't know what else to tell you. This testicle is too far gone to ever make sperm again."

"Doctor, there must be something you can do! Can't you collect sperm from the testicle before you remove it? Aren't there sperm still inside?"

I must say, I felt compassion for Patrick. What man hasn't done something really, really dumb at some point in his life to try to win the favor of a woman?

"Patrick, I don't know if it's possible to find any sperm. I sincerely doubt it. However, it is true that there have been some remarkable advances in fertility treatment. Nowadays, we can help women make babies even with extremely few sperm. If you decide to have the surgery, I can try to find some sperm to collect and freeze when I remove the testicle, but you have to realize it's highly unlikely."

"Doctor, I definitely want the operation if you might save some of my sperm."

The Search for Patrick's Sperm

At surgery, I made an incision in the thickened scrotal skin and quickly found the testicle twisted twice around its blood supply. The testicle was very dark, purple-black. I untwisted it. A few minutes later, its appearance was unchanged. I cut into the testicle. There was no bleeding, as there should have been. The tissue inside was a necrotic soup. The testicle was dead.

Normally, at this point I would have cut the testicle out, sutured the stump so it wouldn't bleed, and closed the wound. However, I had promised Patrick that I would do my best to search for sperm.

I had never been in this situation before, trying to find sperm as the clock ticked on a dying or dead testicle. I thought about what I could do. The testicle itself is the sperm factory, but when I opened Patrick's up there had been no viable tissue, so there was no point in looking for sperm there. From the testicle, the sperm travel first to the epididymis, a series of closely coiled tubes, like miniature angel-hair spaghetti. I cut into the epididymis in several places, but the epididymis also was discolored and dead. No sperm.

From the epididymis, sperm travel into the thicker, more muscular tube called the vas deferens, or "vas" for short. This is the tube that is cut and tied off when a man undergoes a vasectomy. The purpose of the vas is to transport sperm rapidly during ejaculation from the end of the epididymis up into the urethra, the urine passageway, where it mixes with the fluid from the prostate and seminal vesicles to create semen. It is a rather remarkable journey, the equivalent of being shot into space in a rocket ship. Many urologists have their medical students feel the vas, then joke, "And *that* is the vas deferens between men and women."

I decided to go above the level of where the twist had taken place, since the tissues there, including the vas, should have had normal blood supply even during the torsion period. The tissues were indeed pink and obviously healthy, in contrast with the dark tissues below the twist. I opened up the vas deferens at this location, hoping that fluid containing live sperm might still be inside the tube. However, there was none to be found. I massaged the tube above and below the cut, hoping to express a drop or two of fluid, but the well was dry. I was running out of options for Patrick.

As a last-ditch attempt, I took a urethral catheter, passed it from the tip of the penis into the bladder, and emptied out the urine. I then took the smallest intravenous catheter available, designed for infants, and placed it inside the tiny lumen (opening) of the vas. I flushed it with saline toward the abdomen, hoping that any sperm lying along the tube from a previous ejaculation would be washed into the urethra and then the bladder. I passed the catheter into the bladder again, this time collecting the new fluid into a cup. Since I'd just emptied the bladder a moment ago, this new fluid should all have come from what I'd flushed through the vas. This was Patrick's last hope.

I took the cup to a microscope in an adjacent room. I put a drop of the bladder fluid on a slide, placed a glass coverslip over it, and examined the fluid microscopically under medium power. It took a moment to focus, but then I thought I saw something moving. Sperm! There they were, tails going back and forth, some leisurely, some appearing to be in a big hurry. There weren't that many, but I was thrilled for Patrick anyway. I added a special buffer solution to the fluid to preserve the sperm as best I could, and sent it off to the laboratory to be frozen. I returned to the operating room, where I removed the dead testicle and closed the wound.

I went to visit Patrick in the recovery room about an hour later. It was late. Celeste was with him, sweet and tender, holding his hand, stroking his arm.

"How's the pain?" I asked.

Patrick waved off my question. "I'm fine, Doctor. I have no pain. Did you find sperm?"

"Yes," I answered, and Patrick looked visibly relieved. Celeste squeezed his hand. "Not very many. But enough to give you a reasonable chance at creating a pregnancy."

"Thank you, Doctor, thank you so much." This had been the single most important thing for Patrick, the only reason, really, for him to undergo surgery. He was still groggy from the medications, I saw. As he relaxed with the news, his eyes closed, and I watched him drift off to sleep.

Celeste spoke. "Doctor, Patrick told me what had happened. I feel terrible I didn't get him to a doctor while we were in Montreal. I knew he was in pain, but whenever I suggested we go to see a doctor, he refused and told me I was being silly to be concerned about him. I even spoke with the concierge at the hotel about bringing in a doctor, but Patrick wouldn't hear of it."

I shook my head. "Most men with this problem would have taken themselves straight to an emergency room. He told me this trip was very important to him."

Celeste smiled. "He's such a sweet, gentle man. And stubborn, apparently! I'm worried about him, Doctor. Will he be all right?"

"Yes, medically he should be fine. He will have some pain from the incision, but the other pain should be gone already."

"How did you manage to find sperm?" Celeste asked. "That must have been complicated." I explained what I'd done. "That was a lot of work. We both appreciate your efforts. What matters to me most now is that Patrick is all right."

Together with the resident who assisted at the case, I described what we'd done to collect sperm from Patrick and we published it in the *Lancet*. I had fun coming up with the title. We called it "Management of Impending Sterility."

Patrick recovered, and about a year later he and Celeste underwent a cycle of in vitro fertilization to try to have a child with the frozen sperm I'd found. It didn't work. They tried a second time, using up the last of the frozen sperm, and again it didn't work. Sometime afterward Patrick and Celeste broke up. Patrick has continued to see me for testosterone therapy for many years. We've discussed testicular implants for his empty scrotum, but he's not interested.

At Patrick's most recent visit with me, I asked him about that episode of testicular torsion.

"Celeste was the one for me," he said. "I was crazy for her. We clicked on every level. Obviously, I was foolish to not go to the emergency room when I began having pain in the testicle. I knew how dangerous it could be, but all I could think of was that this was my big chance with Celeste, and I needed to be tough enough to see it through. It felt like life and death for me. Now I see how it was so shortsighted of me, because my 'toughness' to be with her that weekend led to my having no chance to marry her."

"Why do you say that?" I asked.

"Celeste wanted to be a mother, to have a family," Patrick answered evenly. "She loved me. I know she did. When the IVF cycles failed, though, and there was no more of my sperm remaining, it was a very difficult time for us. She wanted to get pregnant, and there was nothing I could offer her."

"What about using donor sperm?" I asked. "Or adoption. Did you consider that?"

"The infertility doctors talked to us about it. I was all for it. I would have done anything to be with her. Celeste said it was wrong, though. She didn't want to have a baby using sperm from someone she didn't know and love. She believed that if it wasn't possible for us to have our own children together, then maybe we weren't meant for each other."

"Do you still keep in touch?"

"She married someone else and had a baby within fifteen months. She used to send me a Christmas card every year with a picture of the baby, but I haven't heard from her now in many years."

"Ouch!"

"I don't think she sent the picture to be mean. She was a proud mother, and she loved that baby. I tell myself that in her heart she wanted me to be the father. I know I do that to make myself feel better."

Patrick has dated a number of women over the years. He never married.

A Sacrifice for Fame

Earlier, I explained why it isn't as risky as once believed to give testosterone to men with prostate cancer. However, the more important contribution of Huggins's work in 1941 was to show that total or near-total elimination of testosterone did cause prostate cancer to regress, at least for a while. As a resident I performed dozens of castrations in men with metastatic prostate cancer, and their bone pain from metastatic disease often improved within hours. The testosterone-prostate cancer story back then was king. Not only were we taught that high testosterone levels made prostate cancer grow and low levels of testosterone were protective, but in any discussion of prostate cancer it was to be expected that one attending urologist or another would point out that if a man were castrated early enough in life he would *never* develop prostate cancer. I remember as a resident asking one of my teachers how this was known about prostate cancer, since it occurred to me there must be very few men who had been castrated as youths. "The castrati," came the answer. "Look it up."

I didn't have time to go to the library to research castrati, so I did the next best thing. I asked my chief resident, Dr. Noel DeFelippo, keeper of all useful knowledge and akin to a god to lower-level residents such as myself at the time.

"The castrati?" he echoed. "The castrati were the Italian choirboys with high voices who were castrated before puberty so their voice didn't deepen. They were famous and traveled the world."

"You're kidding," I said. "Boys would give up their testicles so they could sing?"

"They were famous," Noel explained. "It was an honor to be one of the castrati."

"Some honor," I commented sarcastically. "That meant they could never have sex and could never have a family."

"True, but they came from poor families, and becoming a castrato [the singular of castrati] gave a boy the chance to bring money and fame to his family and community. And they lived well. It's a trade-off. Listen, you and I wouldn't do it, but they did. Anyway, the castrati supposedly never got prostate cancer. That's why urologists care about them."

Many years later while investigating the relationship between testosterone and prostate cancer I finally took the time to look into the castrati. The basics of the castrati story Noel told me were correct. They were most popular in the seventeenth and eighteenth centuries. These men with "angel voices" sang at operas and for the church. Since women were not allowed to perform in those days, the castrati played the female parts. Some of the castrati gained considerable fame, and the castrato Farinelli is considered one of the best opera singers who ever lived. The curious part of the castrati story with regard to prostate cancer was that the last known castrato, Alessandro Moreschi from the Sistine Chapel choir, died in 1922. Testosterone itself wasn't discovered until 1935, and a hormonal relationship between testosterone and prostate cancer wasn't suggested until 1941. So despite medical lore, the castrati could not have had any effect on our knowledge about prostate cancer.

The castrati story was interesting, though, even if it had nothing to do with prostate cancer. The practice was condemned by papal decree in 1878. Since the procedure to become a castrato was against religious and civil law, parents offering up their sons with good voices would say that the testicles had already been injured. Apparently, a common story involved an injury sustained from a wild boar. From descriptions in texts of that time, it appears the testicles were not actually removed. Instead, the spermatic cord in the scrotum that carries the blood supply to the testicles was ligated (tied off), preventing blood from reaching the testicles, just as if the boy had suffered a torsion. The result was two shrunken testicles that did not produce the testosterone to trigger the onset of male puberty, which would enlarge the larynx and produce the deeper voice.

My investigation of the prostate cancer–testosterone link led me to another story of eunuchs. In 1960 a Chinese urologist named Wu and his colleague, Gu, investigated the twenty-six surviving eunuchs of the Qing dynasty in China. In umpteen medical conferences I had heard that none of these elderly eunuchs had prostate cancer, thus seeming to prove the assertion that early castration protected against prostate cancer.

A few years ago I finally got my hands on this article, sent to me by a colleague. It is at once a medical article and a historical treatise. And it explained to me something that had bothered me about the traditional notion of eunuchs from my first days of urology training.

My only knowledge of eunuchs had been that these men had been castrated, that is, had their testicles removed, and were thus considered safe to guard the harems of kings and emperors. This made sense to me until I learned in training that as many as 10 to 20 percent of castrated men were still able to have sex. I'd seen patients myself who were able to do so. If some of these castrated men could still have sex, how could they be trusted with the harem girls? I wondered.

The answer lay in the article by Wu and Gu. These eunuchs were used by the nobility for a variety of servant duties, not just guarding the harems. There had been tens of thousands of them in the heyday of the Qing dynasty. The few surviving eunuchs examined by the investigators all lived in government housing. The oldest was eighty-three and the youngest fifty-nine. Most had undergone surgery to render them eunuchs prior to puberty. Wu and Gu's examination of these eunuchs as older men revealed small prostates in all of them, and in some of them the prostate was too small even to be palpable. This was interesting to read but had no direct connection to prostate cancer, which is not mentioned at all in the article. In fact, there is nothing in this frequently cited article that could prove anything about prostate cancer. There were only twenty-six remaining eunuchs out of a population of many thousands. For all we know, the other thousands could have *all* died of prostate cancer. Neither the castrati nor the Chinese eunuch stories provide any proof whatsoever that low testosterone is protective against prostate cancer. But the stories *seemed* to fit if they weren't examined too closely. Unfortunately, medicine is full of this type of lore. As a colleague likes to say, "Doctors learn from doctors, who learned from other doctors, who learned from other doctors, who learned from some guy who made shit up."

Beyond the prostate cancer story, though, the article by Wu and Gu finally explained why eunuchs were considered safe to guard the harem girls. They had not just been castrated, meaning their testicles were gone. Nope. This was worse—they had been emasculated. Here is the text of the surgical procedure to produce a eunuch, originally published in a 1932 article, and included in the article by Wu and Gu. It is not for the faint of heart.

> The subject is placed in a semi-supine position on a broad bench. One man squatting behind him grasps his waist and another man is to look after the legs. Bandages are fastened tightly around the hypogastric and inguinal regions. The *penis and the scrotum* [emphasis added] are three times bathed in a hot decoction of pepper pods. *All the parts* [emphasis added] are swiftly swept away by one stroke of a sickle-shaped knife, a pewter-plug is inserted into the urethra, and the wound is covered with paper soaked in cold water and is firmly bandaged. For three days he gets nothing to drink nor is the plug removed from the urethra. At the end of this period the dressings are changed and the accumulated urine is allowed to escape. The eunuch requires one hundred days for recovery . . . The pubic region of an eunuch, looking from the front, resembles that of a female . . . The mortality of this operation was said to be 2%. Only the specialist, called a "Knifer," was allowed to perform the operation.

So the reason the eunuchs were safe to guard the harem is that they had neither testicles *nor* a penis. I'd never known this critical detail.

An Ounce of Virility from Whatever Source Available

The connection between the testicles and virility has been recognized for millennia, but beginning in the nineteenth century, the testicles and their function became the focus of the search for the "fountain of youth" for men.

On June 1, 1889, Charles-Edouard Brown-Séquard, a prominent French physiologist, announced at the Société de Biologie in Paris that he had developed a therapy for the rejuvenation of the body and mind by creating an extract from the testicles of dogs and guinea pigs. Following a grand tradition in medicine, he had used himself as his first subject. In a paper published in the *Lancet* the next month, he wrote, "I am seventy-two years old. My general strength, which has been considerable, has notably and gradually diminished during the last ten or twelve years. Before May 15th last, I was so weak that I was always compelled to sit down after half an hour's work in the laboratory . . . For many years, on returning home in a carriage by six o'clock after several hours passed in the laboratory, I was so extremely tired that I invariably had to go to bed after having hastily taken a very small amount of food.

"The day after the first subcutaneous injection, and still more after the two succeeding ones, a radical change took place in me, and I had ample reason to say and to write that I had regained at least all the strength I possessed a good many years ago." Brown-Séquard also reported that not only did his strength increase, but his constipation resolved and the arc of his urine was improved! Brown-Séquard went on to treat many men with his injections.

Eugen Steinach, a Viennese physiologist, came up with another idea to improve virility. He believed that the loss of testicular fluid with ejaculation diminished a man's male "powers," and so in 1918 developed a procedure in which he ligated the "spermatic ducts," that is, the vas deferens. The underlying concept is akin to the recommendation that professional athletes, most notably soccer players, abstain from sex during the day prior to a match, so that they do not lose their "chi." The Steinach operation, as it was known, was said to restore youth and vitality, and for the next two decades this procedure was very popular. According to published reports, celebrity clientele who underwent this procedure included Sigmund Freud and the Nobel Prize–winning poet William Butler Yeats. Yeats claimed he underwent "a strange second puberty" after the Steinach procedure, leading to publication of some of his best poems.

Serge Voronoff, a Russian émigré who studied medicine in

Paris, is credited with being the first person to officially transplant testicular tissue from a monkey into a human, in 1920. Voronoff claimed that the transplanted monkey testicle enhanced a man's virility, and he became known as "the famous doctor who inserts monkey glands into millionaires."

The United States was not immune to this burgeoning interest in renewed male vitality derived from testicles of young animals—and, believe it or not, from those of young humans. In the early twentieth century, Leo Stanley was the resident physician of San Quentin prison in California, In 1918 he began transplanting testicles removed from recently executed prisoners into other inmates of various ages, some of whom reportedly recovered sexual potency. In 1920 the "scarcity of human material" prompted Dr. Stanley to substitute testicles from other animals—ram, goat, deer, and boar—in his transplantation experiments in humans. He performed hundreds of operations, with alleged improvement in symptoms of problems as varied as epilepsy, gangrene, senility, and tuberculosis.

The most colorful of the American sex gland transplantation gurus was Dr. John Brinkley, who attended medical school but never completed his training. Instead, he bought a medical diploma from Kansas City Eclectic Medical University in 1915, and by 1917 had established a medical practice in Milford, Kansas. Brinkley took advantage of the interest in the work of Voronoff and Stein-ach, and developed his own procedure in which he proclaimed he improved sexual function in men by transplanting pieces of goat testicles into the scrotum of humans. He became a preacher and set up a radio station, KFKB, where he lectured on his rejuvena-tion therapies as well as religion.

A story on Dr. Brinkley from the *New York Evening Journal* is captioned "How a famous surgeon combines old-time religion and new-fangled operations on a strange medico-gospel farm." In the middle of the page is a picture of a goat's head, with two "horns" of text. One side reads, "Preaches fundamentalism," and the other side reads, "Practices goat-gland science."

These procedures fell out of favor as medical societies denounced them as ineffectual and many of the practitioners unscrupulous. From numerous transplant experiments, we know today that xenografts (tissue transplanted from one species into another) do not survive because the immune system recognizes the new tissue as foreign and destroys it. Even human-to-human transplants don't survive without immunosuppression, except for identical twins, who are essentially biological clones of each other. So as a long-term treatment, it is clear that none of these transplant procedures could have worked. It does seem possible to me, though, that some of these men may have experienced a transient benefit from testosterone within the testicles of these other animals. That benefit would have been short-lived, perhaps for a few days at most, but might have been enough to create a more positive outlook for those men and the belief that they were improved.

Whatever the reality, one cannot dismiss the importance of testicles to a man's sense of his masculine self. From James Bond to John Wayne to whoever is the latest, greatest, most manly man of them all, we pay them the ultimate compliment, at once recognizing what is the true seat of a man's power, when we say, "That guy has balls."

13. NARCISSUS AND
THE PENIS REFLECTED

Integrity simply means not violating one's own identity.

—ERICH FROMM (1900–1980),
American (German-born) psychoanalyst

In medical school, we were taught to ask a single nonjudgmental sexual question whenever taking a medical history: "Are your sexual partners male, female, or both?" I dutifully asked this question as a medical student even though I found its intrusiveness more embarrassing than my patients seemed to, and documented the answer in my required reports with equal weight as whether the patient smoked or was currently experiencing double vision.

At the time, starting out on my own as a doctor, I knew little about gay men and sex other than what I had picked up from books and movies. In college around 1976 I had taken a girlfriend to a movie at the local art house based on a good review (three stars), without actually reading the review itself. The house was packed, and I was pleased to find two great seats in the center of the theater. It didn't take long, though, to realize this was not just another indie-type movie once the leather-and-chain-clad male actors began groping and French-kissing each other. We stayed for a few eye-opening minutes before making an awkward exit. If this was the gay world, it appeared very different from my own.

Today, homosexuality is one of our most divisive social issues. In most urban centers in the United States, particularly on the east and west coasts, there has been a gradual acceptance of gay and lesbian culture. However, there remains strong antigay sentiment from multiple sources. Apart from the moralistic denigration of homosexuality, there is a widespread belief that men who are gay or who just act or look gay are less manly. Among children in middle school, one of the most insulting things one boy can say to another is "You're a homo" or "Faggot!"

There have been enormous strides toward acceptance of same-sex couples in the United States, with nine states and the District of Columbia having laws permitting same-sex marriage as of 2012. However, these laws are quite recent. Not until 2003 did the U.S. Supreme Court strike down antisodomy laws that made male-male sex a crime against the state, in *Lawrence v. Texas.* Around the world, approximately seventy countries have laws forbidding sexual acts by same-sex couples. In some of those countries it is a crime punishable by death; in others, such as Barbados and Guyana, by life imprisonment.

Laws against homosexuality go back as far as the Middle Assyrian Law Codes in 1075 BC, which state, "If a man has intercourse with his brother-in-arms, they shall turn him into a eunuch." This is the first known edict against homosexuality in the military, a great-great-great grandfather to the policy of "Don't ask, don't tell." Henry VIII introduced the first legislation under English criminal law against sodomy with the Buggery Act of 1533, making buggery (anal intercourse with a man, woman, or animal) punishable by hanging, a penalty not lifted until 1861.

The prevalence of homosexuality has been a topic of great interest within sexual research as well. In the 1980s several studies in the United States and other developed countries suggested that approximately 1 percent of the male population was homosexual. Today's figures are higher, probably due to there being less of a stigma associated with being open about being gay. The latest available data from 2011 indicate that between 3.5 and 4.1 percent of Americans self-identify as gay or lesbian. Other studies focused primarily on gay men put the figure somewhere between 5 and 10 percent. Census data have shown that gay men or women live in every single congressional district in the United States. However, there is a higher concentration in the cities (e.g., 15 percent in San Francisco, 12 percent in Seattle and Boston). Although data indicate that only 6 percent of the New York City population is gay, this still represents the largest population of gays in the country due to the size of the city.

One may believe male-male sex is wrong—immoral, unnatural, repellent—but facts are facts: a great many men are sexually attracted to other men. As one of my friends put it, if a bit crudely, "Your dick knows exactly what it likes." Male homosexuality is not a recent phenomenon, and it did not appear out of the blue due to a sudden decline in morality. In Kinsey's pioneering research in 1948, he reported that 37 percent of men in the United States had achieved orgasm at least once with another male.

Homosexuality may be the "hot" sexual topic in America today, but around the world, and in recent U.S. history, there has been no shortage of sexual practices that have precipitated strong prohibitions and punishments. In tribal Muslim communities in Pakistan and Afghanistan, single women may still be stoned to death for the crime of finding themselves alone with a man who is not a family member. In the United States we may feel smugly immune to such antiquated, intolerant attitudes, yet many readers of this book remember when African American men were lynched for the mere suspicion that they had said, done, or even thought of something of a sexual nature with a white woman. Fear and sexuality are a highly volatile mixture.

Today's sexual battleground is gay sex. My hope is that antigay sentiment will soon be seen through the long lens of history as nothing more than one more intolerant attitude toward sexuality that was discarded as we became more educated about the human condition.

Anatomy as Fine Art

Sean was a forty-seven-year-old gay man in a stable, loving relationship with Lloyd, thirty-eight. They were devoted and monogamous, and had lived together for the past two years. Sean came to see me for a very specific issue: he had begun to soften immediately and completely after orgasm and wanted to know what he could do about this change in his sexual performance.

I explained that it was normal as a man aged for his penis to soften more completely after orgasm, and reassured Sean that this change he'd observed shouldn't affect his ability to have sex in any way.

Sean became increasingly agitated despite my attempts to reassure him. "Doctor," he finally blurted out, "you don't understand. Lloyd is a lot younger than I am. He's cute, smart, and successful. Lloyd could be with a lot of guys, but he's with me. One thing he's always appreciated about me is my cock, and it's making me very nervous that it doesn't look or act the way it's supposed to."

"Are you saying you believe Lloyd is with you because of your penis?" I asked.

Sean nodded affirmatively. "It's magnificent when it's hard. Great girth and length, regular coloring, not too veiny. Lloyd calls it the Botticelli of boners," he said with obvious pride. And then his face fell. "He hasn't said that in months," he added.

Like any man or woman, Sean had self-doubts. However, gay men have a set of challenges all their own. In a heterosexual relationship, only one of the partners owns a penis or vagina. There is no basis for comparison or competition. By being experts in their own equipment, gay men are automatically experts in their partner's equipment too. There may be individual preferences and minor differences between individuals, of course, but the basic equipment is the same.

The gay community places a great emphasis on body image, especially on the appearance of the penis, and just like many of the other men discussed in this book, Sean equated his appeal to Alexander with the perceived beauty of his erect penis.

I spoke at length with Sean about what was normal, and tried to reassure him it seemed unlikely that Lloyd would be dissatisfied with him just because his penis softened after orgasm. Sean wouldn't hear of it, though.

"I don't mean to be rude, Doctor," he said, "but you're straight, right?"

"Yes," I answered.

"You just can't understand, then," he concluded, rolling his eyes.

"Maybe not. But it seems to me that if a man's partner is only interested in him because of what his penis looks like, then that's not much of a relationship."

"Well, Doc, that's the relationship I've got. Don't you think Viagra might keep me hard after I come? How about prescribing that for me?"

"I'm sorry, Sean, but I'm not comfortable prescribing Viagra for you. From where I stand, you're normal. Has Lloyd said anything that made you feel this way?"

"No."

"Then my guess would be this is only a problem in your own mind. If Lloyd cares about you, this should be a nonissue."

"No Viagra?" Sean asked again.

"I'm afraid not," I replied.

Sean stood up, shook my hand, and walked silently out the door.

The Male G-Spot

One of the great mysteries in the world of sexuality is the location of the G-spot, the alleged source of uniquely intense and pleasurable sensation in a woman's vagina. The G-spot is named after Ernst Gräfenberg, a gynecologist from New York who published an article in 1950 on the role of the urethra in female orgasm. Sex experts in the early 1980s began referring to an area two to three inches inside the vaginal opening, on the upper surface, as the Gräfenberg zone, which was soon popularized in the popular media as the G-spot. Whether or not the G-spot exists is controversial, as a generation of sex researchers and anatomists have searched for it with little conclusive success. Yet there are many G-spot believers, who claim that stimulation of this area provides mind-blowing orgasms for women. A twist on this controversy is the idea that men have their own G-spot, namely the prostate. Stimulation of the prostate during anal intercourse or by anal insertion of a finger or dildo is said to provide a man with an intense orgasm that can't be replicated by any other kind of stimulation.

The prostate is about the size of a golf ball and sits at the base of the bladder. The urethra runs through the middle of it, like the hole in a bagel, on its way through the penis and out the tip. The function of the prostate is to contribute one or two milliliters of fluid to the semen during ejaculation. Medically, the prostate is important because it often grows with age, causing urinary symptoms well known to older men, such as a weaker stream and more frequent and urgent urination. The prostate can also become inflamed (prostatitis) and cancerous. The only way a doctor can examine the prostate is by inserting a gloved finger into the rectum and feeling frontward.

A straight friend asked me once, "Since gay guys find anal sex so pleasurable, is anal stimulation for the guy something that straight couples should do more? Are we missing out on a great experience?"

The pleasure of anal sex is not all about the prostate. Women who engage in anal sex enjoy it, and they don't have a prostate like men. The pleasure comes from stimulation of the exquisitely sensitive anal area, and from the role play of submission, that taps into deep parts of our brains.

I don't doubt that some men find the experience of prostate stimulation fantastic, but it's hard for me to believe it is a universally amazing experience. I've never seen anyone get hard, ever, from a rectal examination of the prostate.

So is the prostate the male G-spot? Not in my book. Indeed, many men find it uncomfortable, unpleasant, and even painful to have anything inserted into their anus. I consider the prostate just one more part of the body that when stimulated feels great for some men and not others.

Tops and Bottoms

Early in my career, I met Frank, forty-eight, a fund manager at a major investment firm in the Boston area, who said, like many of my patients before and since, "My erections aren't hard anymore." He described how they gradually lost firmness over the previous two years and noted that he no longer experienced morning erections.

After I went through a series of my standard questions, I asked, "Are your partners male or female?"

Frank smiled at me as if he'd been through this generic questioning before and replied, "I'm gay, Doctor." He was making it easy for me and filled me in on the details.

Frank had been with Grant, fifty-two, for eleven years. They were monogamous and were both HIV negative. There was nothing about Frank that would have given me any clue he was gay, and I said so.

"Good!" he replied. "The world of investment banking is pretty macho. My friends know I'm gay, and my parents do too. But no one at work knows." Frank and Grant attended social events together but not business-related ones. "I try to avoid those," he said. "Someone is always trying to set me up with their daughter or sister."

"So how does the weaker erection affect your sex life?" I asked.

Frank looked at me as if this were an exceedingly odd question, and though the answer may have been obvious to Frank, it wasn't obvious to me. For straight couples, a weak erection means the man can't have sex in the usual way with his partner, penis inside vagina. But what did it mean for a gay couple?

"Well, it's difficult to have sex," he said cautiously.

"What part of it is difficult?" I asked.

Frank shifted in his seat and screwed up his face awkwardly.

"I'm not trying to embarrass you, Frank. I'm just trying to understand, because every man is different. Tell me, are you able to have an orgasm?"

"Yeah, sure."

"It feels good?"

"It feels great. There's no problem there."

"Your desire for sex, the hunger for it, is still strong?"

"Yes."

"And do you practice anal sex with Grant?"

"Well, I used to until this problem developed."

It is a misconception that all gay men engage in anal sex. Data from the National Institutes of Health indicate that approximately two-thirds of gay men have experienced anal intercourse at some time, and a smaller number do it routinely. Oral sex and mutual masturbation are more common. Another misconception is that anal sex is only for gay men. Approximately 10 percent of straight couples engage in anal sex as a routine part of their sexual repertoire, usually with the man entering the woman. This means that at any given moment in time there are more straight couples engaging in anal sex than gay men.

"Is anal sex what's difficult now?" I asked.

"Yeah," Frank answered. "Grant likes anal sex. He's a bottom. That works fine for me, since I'm a top. But it's tough to be a top when you can't get hard enough to penetrate."

Now we were getting to the root of the issue.

"Frank," I said, "what do you and Grant do sexually now that you're not able to go inside?"

"We do other stuff, but it's not the same. We've tried toys, but it's not the same."

"What do you mean by 'toys'?"

"You know. Dildos. Butt plugs. We tried all sorts of stuff. I insert them into his anus instead of using my penis. Grant felt funny about it, though, because he didn't think I was getting any pleasure out of it. It was a catch-22. I wanted to give him pleasure, but he wouldn't let me because he thought it wasn't pleasurable for me."

"What about switching roles for anal sex?"

Frank smiled at me and said, "It doesn't work that way, Doctor. Most tops are always tops, and the same goes for bottoms. Some guys do it both ways. We call them 'versatile.' But the joke in the gay community is that when someone calls himself 'versatile,' it means he was a top—one time. Truth is, I don't care for it the other way. It's not a dominance thing, like some people say. It's just unpleasant for me."

"How has your relationship been affected by this?"

"We're not as close. I don't know if it's because I feel bad because I'm not holding up my end of the bargain, or if it's because Grant is pissed off at me. Every year we would go to Napa for a week of wine, friends, and fun. We'd plan it and talk about it for months beforehand, but this year we never got around to booking the trip. We haven't done a weekend getaway in months, either, and that was something we used to do regularly. We've been monogamous for almost the whole time we've been together, but it wouldn't shock me if Grant started going out again."

Frank's tests showed that his nighttime erections were weak. His physical examination and testosterone levels were normal. Viagra hadn't been invented yet; the most common treatment for ED at the time was the penile injections. I gave Frank a trial injection in the office.

"Whoa!" Frank exclaimed as his penis filled and became fully erect within ten minutes. "This is hard!" he said with pleasure and relief.

Frank learned to do the injections himself, and I saw him two months later. "The injections work great," he reported. "I never thought I'd ever be sticking a needle into my penis, but it doesn't hurt at all."

"That's great," I said. "How's the relationship going these days?"

Frank smiled. "Grant and I have reconnected. Sex was a big part of our lives, and we drifted apart when we weren't doing it as much. It's not just the sex, though. It's everything that goes with it. Grant says I'm more of an asshole these days, but he says it as if it's a compliment." Frank switched gears. "Hey, do you remember the Napa trip we missed last year?"

"Yes."

"Well, next month we're off to France. I convinced Grant it was time to step up our wine game. We've always considered Bordeaux too pricey, but what the heck. You only live once."

Years later, when Massachusetts law was changed to permit gay marriage, Frank and Grant were among the first wave of married couples. I saw Frank back in the office for a routine follow-up. "Congratulations!" I said when Frank told me about his marriage. "I can't help but notice the wedding band. Does that mean you've come out at work now?"

"Not exactly," Frank answered. "It's not as if I took out a billboard to announce it, but I don't pretend anymore. I don't need to. I've started my own firm, together with a guy in the business I've known for years. He's straight. When we talked about doing this, I told him I was gay, married actually. He said it didn't matter to him. So now I'm out."

"What's that like?"

"It was weird at first. I felt like I was continually looking over my shoulder, waiting to run into someone I knew, and there would be an awkward conversation. Now that I've relaxed with it, though, this is the best I've ever felt. I'm happy being married. I never thought it was a big deal, but it is. It normalizes everything. No more double life for me. I'm in my fifties now, and for the first time in my life I feel like I can just be who I am."

The Last to Know

Jared was a forty-seven-year-old man referred to me for absent libido and low T. He was married, with a ten-year-old daughter. It had been seven years or longer, he said, since he'd had sex with his wife. Jared told me their relationship was good, he found her attractive, but he just had no sexual desire, for his wife or anyone else. Jared also had osteoporosis, diagnosed after he broke a bone in his foot after a minor accident. His doctor tested his blood and discovered Jared had low T levels. Jared was referred to me for T therapy, which would be beneficial for his bones and would also hopefully restore his sex drive.

Everyone in my office assumed Jared was gay. When I had first met him and we discussed his low sexual desire, I broached the subject of sexual orientation, saying, "Sometimes low desire can occur when men are trying to figure out what turns them on. I've seen a number of married men who just aren't excited by a female partner."

"Doctor, I'm the last person on this planet who would be gay," Jared said. "I used to have desire for my wife, and now I don't. I don't even masturbate anymore. It's like the desire switch in my head has been turned off." This was a classic description for what other men often experienced when their testosterone levels were low, so I let the sexual orientation issue slide, and we proceeded with a trial of testosterone therapy.

After six months Jared declared his sexual desire was still nil. He came into the office for an injection every two weeks. He took no other medications that might affect his desire, and he staunchly declared he was not depressed. Eventually, when it became clear that T therapy wasn't going to solve his low libido, I explained to Jared that sometimes it's impossible to know why libido disappears in some men. I offered to stop the testosterone therapy, but he continued with it to help with his bone density.

A few years after beginning treatment, Jared raised the libido issue again. I encouraged him to see a psychiatrist. "Sometimes there are deep-seated issues that affect us profoundly that we're not even aware of," I explained.

Jared saw the psychiatrist. "Nice guy," he said, "but I didn't find it helpful. And he didn't come up with anything to explain why I have no sexual desire."

A few years later, Jared came in for his regular injection and said, "I have big news for you! Big. You'd better sit down."

"What is it?" I asked.

"I'm gay! Can you believe it? I'm gay. I have a new shrink, and we both realized it—I'm gay."

"Wow! Have you started seeing anyone?"

"No! Are you kidding? How can you even ask me a question like that?"

"Well then, how do you know you're gay?"

"You don't need to have sex with a man to be gay," he lectured, as if explaining the ways of the world to a young child. "It's who I *am*, not what I've done."

"So do you fantasize about men sexually now?"

"I do! It's been so long since I've fantasized about anything! Yes, I fantasize about men now. I'm happy. I feel like I'm finally alive."

Jared saw me for an annual exam several months later. By that time he had had sex with a man. Quite a few, actually. "All those years when I had no libido," he said, "I think it was just suppressed inside me. I wasn't willing or able to recognize it. I think it was psychologically easier for me to have no sexual interest at all than to admit I was turned on by men. I grew up thinking homosexuality was a terrible thing."

"How are things with your wife?" I asked.

"Ruth's been amazing. She says she's not surprised. She says when we stopped having sex all those years ago she was pretty sure this was why. You know what? The marriage worked for all of us. We're divorcing now, and it's a new chapter for all of us. Our daughter, Samantha, went off to college this past year, and she's thriving. She's got a summer internship at a publishing house when her academic year is up, and she talks about living in New York after she graduates."

"Does your daughter know about your big change?"

"Yes. We had a big family meeting when Samantha came home during spring break. She was upset at first when I told her, but she accepts it. She gave me a big hug at the end of our conversation and told me she loved me no matter what, and just wanted me to be happy with who I was."

"It Moved!"

The more a man is worried about his manliness, it seems, the more he needs to be assured he isn't gay. In a classic scene from the television comedy *Seinfeld*, the character George, played by Jason Alexander, winds up at a spa having a massage from a man when no female masseuse is available. Later, George walks into his friend Jerry's apartment, clearly distraught by the idea that he must be gay because of his penis's reaction to massage by a man. "It moved!" he explains to Jerry.

Despite a growing openness about sexuality and the availability of the incredible resources of the Internet, we are still uncertain about so much related to sex. George's fear that he was gay because he developed a partial erection while being massaged captures the sexual uncertainty of many men, and is comical mainly because of George's exaggerated response.

Attack of the "Semi"

Aaron was a forty-seven-year-old gay man who had been partnered with Corey, forty-four, for four years. Aaron was casually dressed in a billowy white linen shirt and expensive-looking pants with great "drape." His dark hair was salt-and-pepper at the temples, and he wore an unusual-looking pair of small rectangular glasses. Aaron was at least twenty pounds overweight, although he wore it well. He took medications for hypertension, diabetes, and high lipid levels. He ran a successful fine art dealership on fashionable Newbury Street in downtown Boston.

"How can I help you?" I asked.

"My penis doesn't get hard anymore," Aaron replied.

"Tell me how this came about."

"It's been going on for about a year. First it was just a bit softer and not always. Now it's never really firm. It just gets semifirm. In fact, that's what my boyfriend, Corey, and I call it: a 'semi.'"

"How's your desire for sex?"

"There's nothing wrong there, Doctor. Everything else seems fine too. I can still have a great orgasm. It's just odd to be nearly soft when it happens, though."

"Do you do anything different sexually now with Corey because you're not as hard?"

"We don't have sex as often, if that's what you're asking."

"Anything else?"

"No."

Aaron and Corey did not engage in anal intercourse. They did when they started out together, but both of them preferred other ways to satisfy each other.

"Since you don't need rigidity to have sex, because you don't need to penetrate," I explained, "I'm wondering how the lack of firmness affects sex for you and Corey."

Aaron nodded in understanding. "It's not about 'doing' anything with it, Doctor. It's about the firmness itself. Who finds a limp dick sexy? Corey is a guy. He knows what a firm penis is— he's got one! You wouldn't believe the fights we've had over my 'semi.' When it started, Corey was sure it was because I didn't find him sexy anymore. He'd put on a bit of weight, as I have, and he was very self-conscious about it. He'd always had a tight, chiseled body, but then he went into a funk when his mother died, and he turned to barrels of Edy's churned cookie dough ice cream as therapy. He thought I was turned off by him, and one time he even accused me of having sex with a longtime friend, who, trust me, I am *not* attracted to.

THE TRUTH ABOUT MEN AND SEX   259

"Anyway, we got past that, and by now Corey knows my 'semi' is *my* problem and has nothing to do with him. My regular doctor explained to him that my diabetes and other medical problems have created this problem for me."

"That's true," I confirmed. "You have a number of health issues that are contributing to your weak erection. Has Corey said that he finds your erection unappealing? Is that what you're concerned about?"

"Not really. Corey can say some nasty things when he's upset, but never about my body or anything having to do with sex. Thank God! Actually, he still treats me the same as he always did when my erection was good. I think it's more about how *I* feel about it. I'm embarrassed by it."

Aaron hesitated before continuing. "You know, my relationship with Corey is great, but we do have some awful fights sometimes, and when we do, I can't help but think about being out there on my own again. That thought gets me really depressed. How could I ever find anyone with my limp member? Just to be clear, I'm not interested in leaving Corey. Not at all. I guess what I'm saying is that it makes me feel pathetic to be this way."

I prescribed daily low-dose Cialis for Aaron. When it works, it's an excellent solution for many men. The main drawback is that health insurance usually doesn't pay for more than four or six pills per month, so a daily dose can be expensive. Aaron was willing to pay for it.

When he came back for a follow-up after six weeks, I asked how things were going.

Aaron was all smiles. "The Cialis works great," he told me. "Corey and I are doing really well."

"I'm so happy to hear that," I said.

"You know, Doctor, when I first saw you, I didn't really get it when you asked me how my weak erection affected me. Now that my erection is firmer, I find I think about sex more. I have more confidence. Sex is more fun. I play around with Corey more, and frankly, I find that I flirt with people again outside of work. Even with women, sometimes! Why not?" He shrugged his shoulders, as if to say, "I can't help myself!"

"That's really interesting," I replied.

Aaron continued. "It's amazing how much of sex is in the head. The short answer to your question is that I don't *do* anything different with a hard penis than I did with a soft one, but the entire experience for me has changed. I'm a different person. I can't believe a hard penis makes me happy, but there it is."

"Don't be so rough on yourself," I said. "You're not alone with this. Nearly every man who comes through my office feels better about himself if he can get a good erection. Having a hard penis affects a man's self-esteem, his sense of manliness, and everything else seems to follows from that."

"Well, that makes me feel a bit better. Doctor, I don't think I mentioned this when I saw you before, but I've been in psychotherapy for years with an excellent psychologist. When my erections began to weaken, we explored all sorts of angles about why I wanted sex less and why I was feeling less sexy. My therapist assigned "homework assignments" for Corey and me, and some of them were a bit helpful. However, none came close to making me feel as good as having a hard penis. I pay a lot for the Cialis you prescribed, but it's still a heck of a lot cheaper, and more effective, than those sessions with my shrink!"

14. MEN ARE PEOPLE TOO!

The American ideal of sexuality appears to be rooted in the American ideal of masculinity. This idea has created cowboys and Indians, good guys and bad guys, punks and studs, tough guys and softies, butch and faggot, black and white. It is an ideal so paralytically infantile that it is virtually forbidden—as an unpatriotic act—that the American boy evolve into the complexity of manhood.

—JAMES BALDWIN (1924–87), American writer

Every day for almost twenty-five years men of all stripes have passed through my exam room, often accompanied by their partners, sharing with me their most intimate problems. Behind the closed doors of my office I have had the rarest of opportunities: to listen to men speak about a secret part of human experience. The discussions I've had with men about sex are usually the only discussions those men have had in that kind of detail, anywhere. This world of male sexuality, full of surprises, twists, and emotions, has made me repeatedly reassess my own thoughts and beliefs as to what men are all about. In this book I have attempted to pull back the curtain for my readers—male and female—providing access to this precious material in order to reveal men as they really are.

The absurd overemphasis on men's libido as the ultimate descriptor of men reminds me of the story of the blind men feeling an elephant. One feels a tusk, another the trunk, another the ear, and still another a leg. Each is convinced he knows what an elephant is like based on the part he examined, but none can adequately describe the elephant as a whole. Somehow our culture lost sight of the fact that with maturity men find themselves interested in far more than sex.

"Yeah, right!" comes the line from the female stand-up comedian. "Of course men are interested in more than just sex. They're also interested in pizza, beer, and football. Whoopee-doo!"

What I see are men trying as hard as they can to do the right thing while pulled in various directions by any number of powerful vectors, including a hormonally driven sexual desire, a search for love, an effort to be "manly," concern about what is socially acceptable, a fear of inadequacy, a desire for power, riches, and respect, to name just a few. Boys may be simple, but men are complex. Men don't always get it right in relationships, but the more I listen to their stories, the more I hear how much the majority of men wish to do well by their partners.

The case that gave rise to the title of this book is a perfect example. When I told friends and colleagues about a young male patient who faked his orgasms, the conversations followed a predictable course. It seemed as if everyone who heard the story resisted it, often with considerable emotion, particularly women. One woman told me outright, "I don't believe you. I think you're making it up."

A woman fakes an orgasm to bring the sexual activities to a socially acceptable end ("He would have kept going forever if I hadn't faked it") and to make her partner feel all right about himself ("I wanted to make him feel good"). Why would a man fake an orgasm? *For exactly the same reasons.*

David loved his girlfriend, Sarah, and began faking his orgasms once he sensed Sarah was becoming concerned she was sexually inadequate. David recognized that faking it entailed significant risk on his part, since he was convinced Sarah would be done with him if she found out.

David's motives are not at all rare. Indeed, listening to the stories of men, one soon discovers that providing pleasure to one's partner is paramount to a man's sexual experience; in many cases, that means giving her full sexual satisfaction, but in some cases, it means making her feel as though she's a great sex partner herself. In fact, providing pleasure for the woman is the measure by which a man determines his manliness. What I never would have guessed when I first started out in the field was how important it is for a man's sense of self to be able to view himself as a good sexual provider.

In order to feel like a good sexual provider, my patient Duncan, a paraplegic, learned to inject his penis so he could have sex with his wife, Janet, even though he didn't feel a blessed thing. Duncan's pleasure came exclusively from being able to provide Janet with enough stimulation so that she could experience sexual satisfaction with his penis inside her. It made him feel manly, whole, to make his wife happy that way.

Many other patients have shown the same concern. The focus on the partner's pleasure and satisfaction as the measure of one's manliness is exemplified by what we call premature ejaculation, which is itself a pejorative, sexist, and anti-male term. Consider: A woman who climaxes during foreplay, prior to intercourse and without direct genital stimulation, would be described in positive terms, as highly responsive, and the man who was fortunate enough to produce this experience for a woman would feel like he is the sexiest man alive. No one would think to label the woman's orgasm as "premature."

Yet the man who unintentionally comes in his pants while making out is open to ridicule. "What a tool!" his own friends might say if they heard about it. "I can't believe he couldn't even hold off long enough to get it in!" Women might have an even harsher description that would question his masculinity. Yet why should we expect a man to "hold off" on the pleasurable experience of an orgasm and not expect the same of a woman? It is because the man who climaxes too soon has failed in what is regarded as his manly role in the dance of sex. An orgasm may be the most pleasurable sensation known to humankind, but trust me when I tell you that men who come too quickly experience no pleasure in the act. They are too busy cursing themselves.

Along these lines, a man who climaxes within thirty seconds of insertion will usually feel fine about himself if his partner can also have an orgasm during that time, whereas a man who lasts thirty minutes but fails to bring his girlfriend to orgasm may feel disappointed in himself even if he successfully accomplished twenty-five Kama Sutra positions. As I've noted before, a man's definition of *great sex* is when the partner says, "That was great sex." One of the great lies of modern sexuality is that men are preoccupied with their own pleasure. The truth is, most men are consumed with providing pleasure to their partner.

It is difficult to be a man these days, and it is no easier within the realm of sexual relations. The roles of men in society, within relationships, and within the family have changed radically over the last forty years. For the first time in U.S. history, a majority of young women giving birth are single mothers. Once upon a time, men had much greater access to sexual information (and to sex) than women, but that's no longer true either. Now we see articles written by professional women in their thirties asking, "What do I need a man for?"

It is difficult these days for a man to figure out what he brings to the party for the modern woman who appears to have everything: career, money, independence, friends. The one obvious thing he can provide is a hard penis. The good part is that it's true that women cannot supply this on their own. The scary part is that the hard penis can be an unreliable resource. Sometimes it's shy and doesn't want to come out to play. Sometimes it starts out all right and then disappears mid-act. And eventually with age and/or illness, in nearly all men the ability to "provide" the hard penis fades away entirely.

The times clearly are a'changing, and it will be interesting to see how the ongoing shift toward female power and autonomy plays out in the world of male/female relationships. Men may feel discouraged by these societal shifts, but I'm confident there will always be an important role for men in the world of relationships. The last time I checked, most women still like men, and most men still like women. We'll muddle through and figure this out eventually.

Sex remains the last taboo. We may be surrounded by sexual imagery on television, in movies and magazines, and bombarded with it on the Internet, but none of this diminishes the mystery, confusion, shame, and unspeakable urges that are associated with it. There is no question that the average sixteen-year-old boy or girl of today knows more about the technical aspects of sex than one from a generation ago—the anatomy, positions, sex toys, et cetera—but I strongly doubt that these kids know anything more about how sex fits into our lives and relationships.

There is no training in sexuality. No education about the psychological nitty-gritty of it. We may learn in sex ed about the penis entering the vagina and about pregnancy and sexually transmitted diseases, but that level of factual information is as far as it goes. Everything else about sex (and sometimes even the basics) is too much of a hot potato to be taken up in school. And once we're out of school, that's it, we're on our own. Since men feel so vulnerable about their masculinity, and since being sexually successful is so critical to feeling okay about one's masculinity, it is extremely difficult for a man to tell his good buddy he can't get it up with his girlfriend or that he comes within ten seconds of inserting his penis in her vagina. And pornography does nothing to teach a man about what sex is supposed to be like. Normal women don't have breasts that large, normal men don't have penises that large, and male porn stars aren't depicted experiencing ED, premature ejaculation, or lack of desire.

The comedian Rodney Dangerfield said, "The first time I had sex I was scared. It was dark. I didn't know what I was doing. *I was alone.*" We are all like Rodney. Our first sexual thoughts and urges were private and terrifically strange. Most of us never mentioned them to friends or parents, and those who did speak up were usually "shushed," shamed, or ridiculed. The truth is that most men and women not only begin their sexual lives in private but continue to live that way, alone and in the dark, forever.

There is another reason most people never speak openly about sex: sex is totally bizarre. There is nothing in human experience like it.

With sex we do intimate, deeply personal, secret things with people we barely know that we never do with friends or family—all the people we know best. We behave this way because as humans we are biologically designed to behave this way. The primitive reptilian part of our brain creates the primal urge to mate. That urge is innate. We may *wish* our sexuality were bounded by reason, logic, and practical considerations, but let's face it—sex is irrational. The drive comes from the deeper part of the brain that deals with things automatically, without conscious thought, which resides in the "newer," more superficial portion of the brain, the cerebral cortex.

Humans are like all other animals with respect to their sex drive. It is arguably the most powerful biological drive of all. Male salmon stop eating and their intestinal system atrophies as they mill about in mating pools at the base of streams, undergoing dramatic bodily changes that prepare them for the upstream trek to spawn—and then they die. The male praying mantis has his head eaten off by the female while they're mating, for cryin' out loud! Sex drive can trump even the basic instincts of self-preservation and survival.

However, unlike other animals (we surmise), the highly developed brain of humans is capable of self-consciousness and reflection. This makes sex a more complicated part of our lives and our sense of self. It also creates a tension in our sexual behavior between our sexual urges and our conscious thoughts, which attempt to provide rationalizations about how sex is supposed to occur. This higher level of consciousness is a gift that allows us to mentally explore primal physical phenomena, like sex, but also creates anxieties and difficulties that are (again, we assume) foreign to other animals.

A poorly recognized additional challenge for men is that sexual problems are so common. The medical field was shocked by the response to a simple question posed by the Massachusetts Male Aging Study in 1994. Among relatively healthy men between the ages of forty and seventy, slightly more than half stated they had some degree of erectile dysfunction. Until then, no one had imagined the number of men dealing with erection problems was that high. Just as surprising was the rate of premature ejaculation, which in contrast to ED affects young men as much as older men, with most studies reporting rates of between 15 and 25 percent of respondents.

Declining levels of testosterone take their toll on men, sexually and in other ways that affect a man's sense of virility and vitality. The resulting "male menopause" may not be universal, but it sure is common as we get into our fifties and beyond. Based on blood results, some studies suggest 40 percent of men or greater experience male menopause after the age of fifty. Peyronie's disease, which causes penile deformity and an abnormally curved erection due to scarring of the tunica albuginea, has been estimated to affect 2 to 5 percent of men. Any number of prescription medications can cause sexual side effects such as ED, diminished libido, and even the inability to achieve an orgasm at all. Prominent among those are the ubiquitous antidepressants known as selective serotonin reuptake inhibitors, or SSRIs.

One of the most common types of medications used to treat the frequent urination and slow stream caused by an enlarged prostate—called alpha adrenergic blockers, with suggestive names like Flomax and Rapaflo—can cause retrograde ejaculation in 20 percent or more of patients. This means semen goes backward into the bladder and then comes out the next time the man urinates. Not technically what we call a sexual dysfunction but certainly a weird experience for the affected man. Put all these numbers together, and that's a lot of men having sexual problems. It makes one wonder if there is any such thing as "normal" sex.

It is a disheartening list of maladies that man is heir to. So let's all give a cheer for the current and approaching set of medical remedies, allowing men to preserve their sexual dignity and power. Men should be grateful to the weird and wonderful demonstration of Dr. Giles Brindley, who scandalously dropped his trousers at a medical meeting, dramatically beginning the modern era of male sexual medicine while also providing a quick kick in the butt to the ideas of Masters and Johnson, who had bollixed up the sex lives of an entire generation of men by authoritatively asserting that impotence was almost invariably caused by psychological problems. Today we have pills that help men get it up and keep it up, and that can even slow down ejaculation. And as the fear recedes that testosterone therapy will cause an epidemic of prostate cancer, there now is a reasonable hope for many men to be sexually active into their twilight years. That's good news for their wives and partners, as well as for the men themselves.

In his book *The Singularity Is Near*, the futurist Raymond Kurzweil predicts that at the current rate of acceleration in technological advancement, by the year 2045 humans will have achieved immortality. That's because technology will be so sophisticated and miniaturized that we will be able to incorporate nanotechnology into our bodies and arrest the aging process at the cellular level. This melding of machine and biology already exists for men with sexual dysfunction, in the form of a penile prosthesis. A cartoon sent to me via e-mail from a colleague shows an open casket with only the tip of an erect penis visible above the edge. We really are sexual creatures from cradle to grave. It will be exciting to see how human sexuality evolves as a result of advances in medicine and technology.

A colleague of mine who lectures on female sexuality likes to show two slides in sequence. The first is the control panel of a machine labeled "Woman." It is a complex picture full of knobs, gauges, rheostats, and slider controls. The second slide is labeled "Man" and appears remarkably simple. The entire control panel is empty apart from a single switch, marked "on" and "off." The audience always laughs, and with these slides my colleague introduces the concept that female sexuality is complex and influenced by many factors. Desire in a woman, she explains, may change moment by moment depending on all the various issues competing for her attention: Is the house clean? Is her period coming? Is lunch made for the kids? What's the status of the presentation due at work on Friday? And so on. By comparison, she says, men are simple and always ready to go. The audience nods their heads in agreement at this obvious comparison with men.

Bullfeathers! It is astonishing to me that our culture has come to an apparent consensus that a man's sex drive is so fixed in place at full throttle that he is impervious to the slings and arrows of daily life. This may be true for a sixteen-year-old, but it's not true for mature men feeling the stress of juggling work and family and personal finances. Believe it or not, sometimes it is the man who declines an invitation for sex. Quite a few men have told me they are incapable of having sex at all when stressed—their equipment simply doesn't respond. If one believes that sex is all a man ever thinks about, no wonder we tend to think of men as simple, lacking in complexity and depth. It is a pervasive attitude, yet false, and it has produced an unnecessary and burdensome obstacle for the creation of loving and respectful relations between men and women.

Men have a set of issues to deal with that are distinct from those of women. As the son of a strong woman and the father of two wonderful daughters, I solidly support the idea that men and women are equal, and I celebrate the fact that women today can create for themselves whatever life they choose. However, political and social equality does not mean men and women are the same. They are not.

One specific issue of central importance to men, especially as they grow into young and middle adulthood, is the struggle to be manly. Men are trained as children to not cry, to not express hurt or sadness, to "be strong." In our culture, men are permitted a more restricted palette of acceptable emotional responses than women. To be tough is to not show emotion. "Real men" don't panic, even in a crisis. They are the ones who are supposed to lead the way out of a collapsed building instead of freaking out at the thought that they might die. It requires training and discipline to suppress one's emotions. I will leave it to others to debate whether or not it's "healthy" for men to deny their emotions. "Manly" stoicism may be admirable in many situations, but today's woman pines for a man who is emotionally available. It is a high-wire act to be able to do both.

In the movie *The Descendants* (2011), the viewer's heart goes out to Matt King (played by George Clooney) as he struggles with his sadness at the imminent death of his wife, despite learning that she had been having an affair and had planned to divorce him. Matt gets his troubled teenage daughter to accompany him on a visit to the wife's family, and she insists on bringing along her boyfriend, a surfer-dude type who seems excruciatingly insensitive with his constant jokes. He is a paragon of the clueless, dumb young male until Matt has a late-night conversation with him in which he learns that the boyfriend's father had died just a few months earlier in a car crash. In an instant, we see the pain behind the clown's mask. The boyfriend's character had seemed to be pure comic relief, but in a small moment that speaks volumes we see that a man's "simple" repertoire of expression may hide a hurt the size of Kentucky.

* * *

One important theme in this book is that most men have the capacity and a strong desire to act nobly. It may be a flawed nobility, as good intentions don't always translate into a successful outcome, but it may still be admirable. Over and over, I see men doing their best to be kind, considerate, and generous to their partners. When we couple good deeds for others with risk, discomfort, or inconvenience for ourselves, that is something to be acknowledged and respected, particularly when it is done with no expectation of anything in return. David, the young man who faked his orgasm, behaved as nobly as he knew how in order to make Sarah feel all right about herself. David didn't strike me as being a do-gooder in other parts of his life, yet in his relationship with the woman he cared for, his behavior was focused on what was best for her.

Not everyone will agree with me about the nature of many men. Women in particular may object to the idea that men are nobler creatures than how they are usually portrayed. One of my friends, a wonderful, highly intelligent woman in her sixties, said to me, "I'm sorry, Abe, but I just don't see it the way you do. Even if a man is intent on pleasing his female partner, isn't that ultimately still selfish rather than noble? Isn't he doing it so that he feels good about himself? It's as if the woman were just the means by which he satisfies his own ego."

I understand the argument, but if you take that point of view, there is no human action that could not be reduced to "He (she) did it because it made him (her) feel good about himself (herself)." I agree that men who think they have done well by their partners sexually feel more manly. However, I reject the argument that it is selfish. Selfish is when a man takes care of himself sexually without any consideration of his partner.

Men also do not necessarily buy into the notion of the noble man. The other day I mentioned my thesis to a longtime patient of mine, a seventy-four-year-old man who had come in for a routine prostate check. "Noble?" He chuckled. "I don't know about that," he said. "My fiftieth wedding anniversary is coming up this year, and although I've never strayed, I've got to be honest, I've never stopped looking at women. And if I had ever found myself in bed with Sophia Loren, who in my day was the Ultimate Woman, I'm pretty sure I would have broken my wedding vows."

It was an interesting conversation, but it didn't sway me. Men feel guilty about their desires. They fantasize about sex with different women. They imagine themselves with movie stars. They feel themselves becoming aroused if an attractive woman flirts with them. Under the right circumstances ("if I had ever found myself in bed with Sophia Loren . . .") they fear they would be unfaithful. In a culture where sexual fidelity is considered the standard, men feel impure just because they may find women other than their partners sexually appealing.

But women have their fantasies too. A former girlfriend gave me her ground rules early in the relationship. "We're each allowed a free pass to sleep with any of five celebrities. I'll give you my list, and you can give me yours," she said generously.

"What do you mean, a free pass?" I asked.

"If I ever meet them, I can sleep with them, and you can't be angry." She went on to list the actors George Clooney and Brad Pitt, the singer Enrique Iglesias, the soccer star David Beckham, and Bibi Netanyahu."

"Netanyahu?" I asked, shocked. "The Israeli politician?"

"I like him," she responded matter of factly. "Anyway, that's my list. Now, who are your five?"

If we are guilty because we feel sexual attraction to someone who is not our partner, then I fear none of us is innocent.

Listening to men over the years has been a mind-opening adventure for me. There is no one-size-fits-all, yet one cannot help but see patterns, trends, and common themes after a while. Is it really such a surprise that when dealing with sex, the most mysterious human activity, men have a set of emotional responses that are complex, nuanced, and profound? Not all men are angels, but there is no shortage of admirable men with noble intentions. These are men who form relationships and care deeply about their partners and the integrity of their bonds. They strive to be good partners, good sons, and good fathers. It is time to reexamine our conventional, misleading negative notions about men so that we may see them as they really are: complex, fascinating individuals, each with a personal story that has brought him to this point in time. I am not a philosopher, but I have come, through this work, to see the goodness in men.

In the end, men are people too. From the very beginning, at birth, we strive to make distinctions between men and women as if they belonged to different species. Some differences do of course exist—differences in upbringing, anatomy, and hormones, among others. However, many readers will be surprised to learn that men and women are as much alike as they are different. And as human beings, we share a connection at our very core: our deepest desire is to find a partner whom we can love and cherish, and who will accept us, and love us back, as we truly are. Recognizing man's true nature through the prism of his sexuality is an opportunity for greater intimacy within relationships and a step toward a greater understanding of our own humanity.

APPENDIX:

DIAGRAMS AND ILLUSTRATIONS

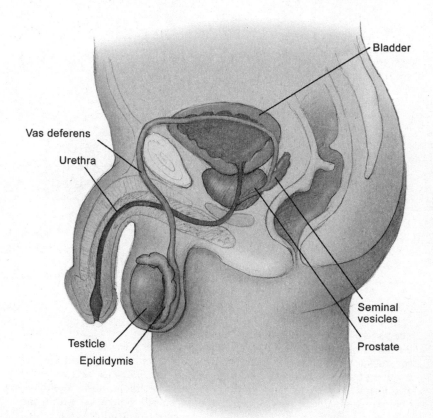

Bladder

Vas deferens

Urethra

Seminal vesicles

Prostate

Testicle

Epididymis

The Male Reproductive System

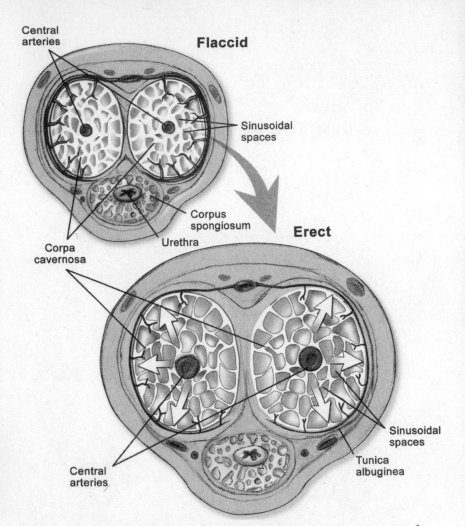

Flaccid

Central arteries

Sinusoidal spaces

Corpus spongiosum

Corpa cavernosa

Urethra

Erect

Sinusoidal spaces

Tunica albuginea

Central arteries

The penis is composed of three cylinders: two paired corpora cavernosa and the corpus spongiosum running on the underside of the penis. The corpora cavernosa are responsible for the firmness of the penis during erection. The corpus spongiosum consists of spongy tissue surrounding the urethra and it also forms the glans, or head, of the penis. With sexual arousal or stimulation, parasympathetic nerves cause smooth muscle relaxation within the corpora cavernosa, resulting in dilation of the cavernosal arteries, which permits delivery of more blood within the corpora cavernosa. The sinusoidal spaces within the corpora cavernosa also expand and compress the veins against the tunica albuginea (the tough sheath surrounding the corpora cavernosa), thus reducing drainage of blood from the corpora cavernosa. This keeps the penis firm. Flaccidity is achieved by sympathetic nerves, which cause constriction of the arteries and sinusoidal spaces, reducing inflow of blood to the penis and allowing blood to exit the corpora cavernosa.

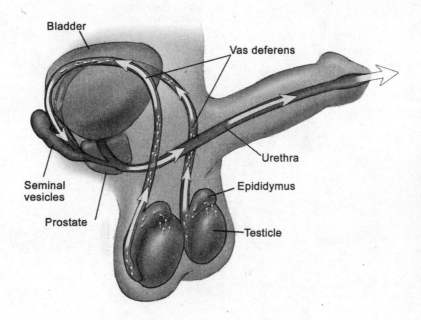

Bladder

Vas deferens

Urethra

Seminal
vesicles

Epididymus

Prostate

Testicle

Sperm produced in the testicles have a long journey before they exit the penis during ejaculation. They first pass through the epididymis, a set of delicate tubes that runs behind the testicle from the top to the bottom. The epididymis then becomes a single, long muscular tube called the vas deferens that transports the sperm during ejaculation. The vas deferens joins the tube from the seminal vesicles, and together they drain into the portion of the urethra lying within the prostate. During ejaculation, sperm and fluid from the testicles are combined with fluid from the seminal vesicles and prostate to create semen. Powerful muscular contractions during ejaculation, controlled by the sympathetic nerves, propel the sperm along its journey and close the opening of the bladder, so that the semen is expelled out the urethra.

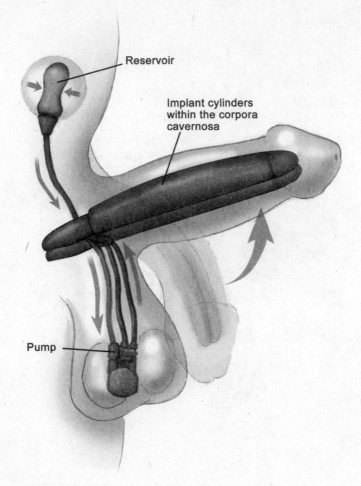

Reservoir

Implant cylinders within the corpora cavernosa

Pump

This figure shows an inflatable three-piece penile implant. Hollow cylinders are placed within the two corpora cavernosa, a reservoir containing saline is placed in the pelvis behind the pubic bone, and a pump is placed within the scrotum. Squeezing the pump in the scrotum inflates the device by transferring fluid from the reservoir in the pelvis to the penile cylinders, which expands and creates an erection. The implant is deflated by pressing a button on the pump, allowing fluid from the penile cylinders to return to the reservoir. Another version is a two-piece implant that replaces the separate reservoir with an area in the rear of the penile cylinders to hold the fluid.

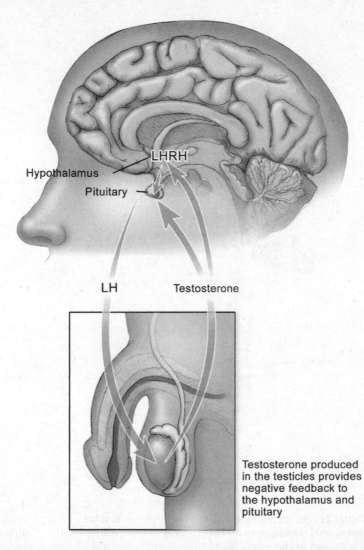

Testosterone produced in the testicles provides negative feedback to the hypothalamus and pituitary

Testosterone in men is primarily produced by the testicles under control of the hypothalamus and pituitary gland in the brain. The hypothalamus sends a chemical signal called luteinizing hormone releasing hormone (LHRH) to the nearby pituitary gland, which in turn releases luteinizing hormone (LH) into the circulation where it eventually reaches the testicles, signaling them to produce testosterone. There is also a negative feedback mechanism governed by concentrations of testosterone in the blood. When testosterone levels are low, more LH is produced to stimulate more testosterone production. When levels are high, LH secretion is reduced until testosterone normalizes.

NOTES

I. INTRODUCTION

7　I would argue: Boston Women's Health Book Collective, *Our Bodies, Ourselves* (New York: Touchstone, 2005).

7　There are other challenges: H. A. Feldman et al., "Impotence and Its Medical and Psychosocial Correlates: Results of the Massachusetts Male Aging Study," *Journal of Urology* 151, no. 1 (January 1994): 54–61.

7　Premature ejaculation affects: H. Porst et al., "The Premature Ejaculation Prevalence and Attitudes (PEPA) Survey: Prevalence, Comorbidities and Professional Help-Seeking," *European Urology* 51 (2007): 816–24; M. Waldinger et al., "A Multinational Population Survey of Intravaginal Ejaculation Latency Time," *Journal of Sexual Medicine* 2 (2005): 292–97; E. O. Laumann et al., "Sexual Problems Among Women and Men Aged 40–80 Y: Prevalence and Correlates Identified in the Global Study of Sexual Attitudes and Behaviors," *International Journal of Impotence Research* 17 (2005): 39–57; T. Mulligan et al., "Prevalence of Hypogonadism in Males Aged at Least 45 Years: The HIM Study," *International Journal of Clinical Practice* 60, no. 7 (July 2006): 762–69.

2. THE MAN WHO FAKED HIS ORGASMS

14　Strange as it may seem: A. Nicolosi et al., "Sexual Activity, Sexual Disorders and Associated Help-Seeking Behavior Among Mature Adults in Five Anglophone Countries from the Global Survey of Sexual Attitudes and Behaviors (GSSAB)," *Journal of Sex and Marital Therapy* 32, no. 4 (July 2006): 331–42.

16   We're familiar with the idea: J. B. Korda, S. W. Goldstein, and F. Sommer, "The History of Female Ejaculation," *Journal of Sexual Medicine* 7, no. 5 (May 2010): 1965–75.

20   Not only do some women: F. Wimpissinger et al., "The Female Prostate Revisited: Perineal Ultrasound and Biochemical Studies of Female Ejaculate," *Journal of Sexual Medicine* 4, no. 5 (September 2007): 1388–93.

22   There can be other: S. Read, M. King, and J. Watson, "Sexual Dysfunction in Primary Medical Care: Prevalence, Characteristics and Detection by the General Practitioner," *Journal of Public Health Medicine* 19, no. 4 (1997): 387–91.

27   For Sylvester: A. Nicolosi et al., "Sexual Behavior and Sexual Dysfunctions after Age 40: The Global Study of Sexual Attitudes and Behaviors," *Urology* 64, no. 5 (November 2004): 991–97.

3. THE FRETFUL PENIS

35   As a rule: A. Morgentaler, "Clinical Crossroads: A 66-year-old Man with Sexual Dysfunction," *Journal of the American Medical Association* 291 (2004): 2994–3003.

38   Normal, healthy men: I. Karacan et al., "Sleep-Related Penile Tumescence As a Function of Age," *American Journal of Psychiatry* 132, no. 9 (September 1975): 932–37; L. A. Levine and R. A. Carroll, "Nocturnal Penile Tumescence and Rigidity in Men Without Complaints of Erectile Dysfunction Using a New Quantitative Analysis Software," *Journal of Urology* 152, no. 4 (October 1994): 1103–7.

4. WHAT IS A MAN?

55   Based on his appearance: E. Chung and G. B. Brock, "Cryptorchidism and Its Impact on Male Fertility: A State of Art Review of Current Literature," *Canadian Urological Association Journal* 5, no. 3 (June 2011): 210–14.

57   Another issue was the increased risk: J. M. Hutson et al., "Cryptorchidism," *Seminars in Pediatric Surgery* 19, no. 3 (August 2010): 215–24.

60   So what happened to Effie?: J. Farikullah et al., "Persistent Müllerian Duct Syndrome: Lessons Learned from Managing a Series of Eight Patients Over a 10-year Period and Review of Literature Regarding Malignant Risk from the Müllerian Remnants," *British Journal of Urology International* (April 30, 2012).

62   Technically, Effie was not: I. A. Aaronson, "True Hermaphroditism: A Review of 41 Cases with Observations on Testicular Histology

and Function," *British Journal of Urology International* 57, no. 6 (December 1985): 775–79.

65 "The technical part of the vasectomy": W. Hsiao et al., "Nomograms to Predict Patency after Microsurgical Vasectomy Reversal," *Journal of Urology* 187, no. 2 (2012): 6.

67 "It could," I answered: S. J. Silber et al., "Pregnancy with Sperm Aspiration from the Proximal Head of the Epididymis: A New Treatment for Congenital Absence of the Vas Deferens," *Fertility and Sterility* 50, no. 3 (September 1988): 525–28.

72 The transgender issue is complicated: N. P. Spack et al., "Children and Adolescents with Gender Identity Disorder Referred to a Pediatric Medical Center," *Pediatrics* 129, no. 3 (March 2012): 418–25.

76 These women were men: O. N. Stern and W. J. Vandervort, "Testicular Feminization in a Male Pseudohermaphrodite, Report of a Case," *New England Journal of Medicine* 254, no. 17 (April 1956): 787–90.

5. A PENIS BY ANY OTHER NAME

82 "It's an operation": M. L. Djordjevic et al., "Metoidioplasty as a Single Stage Sex Reassignment Surgery in Female Transsexuals: Belgrade Experience," *Journal of Sexual Medicine* 6, no. 5 (May 2009): 1306–13.

86 A year earlier: S. Monstrey et al., "Penile Reconstruction: Is the Radial Forearm Flap Really the Standard Technique?" *Plastic Reconstructive Surgery* 124, no. 2 (August 2009): 510–18.

6. BETTER LIVING THROUGH PHARMACOLOGY

96 The *Time* cover story: W. H. Masters and V. E. Johnson, *Human Sexual Inadequacy* (Boston: Little, Brown, 1970).

96 It is hard to overstate: A. C. Kinsey, W. B. Pomeroy, and C. E. Martin, *Sexual Behavior in the Human Male* (Bloomington: Indiana University Press, 1975; first published 1948).

99 It is interesting to look: A. Morgentaler, *The Viagra Myth: The Surprising Impact on Love and Relationships* (San Francisco: Jossey Bass/Wiley, 2003).

99 In the United States today: A. Morgentaler, "Male Impotence," *Lancet* 354 (1999): 1713–18.

102 One older theory: G. G. Conti, R. R. Virag, and W. W. von Niederhäusern, "The Morphological Basis for the Polster Theory of Penile Vascular Regulation," *Acta Anatomica* 133, no. 3 (1988): 209–12.

103 "Before Giles Brindley": I. Goldstein, "The Hour Lecture that Changed Sexual Medicine—the Giles Brindley Injection Story," *Journal of*

Sexual Medicine 9, no. 2 (February 2012): 337–42; L. Klotz, "How (Not) to Communicate New Scientific Information: A Memoir of the Famous Brindley Lecture," *British Journal of Urology International* 96, no. 7 (November 2005): 956–57.

105 Brindley was not the first: R. Virag, "Intracavernous Injection of Papaverine for Erectile Failure," *Lancet* 320, no. 8304 (October 1982): 938.

109 In 1989 I read: G. Wagner, T. Gerstenberg, and R. J. Levin, "Electrical Activity of Corpus Cavernosum During Flaccidity and Erection of the Human Penis: A New Diagnostic Method?" *Journal of Urology* 142, no. 3 (September 1989): 723–25.

7. LISTENING TO VIAGRA

115 Viagra was officially introduced: A. Morgentaler, *The Viagra Myth: The Surprising Impact on Love and Relationships* (San Francisco: Jossey Bass/Wiley, 2003).

124 The way the ED pills work: H. Porst et al., "Efficacy of Tadalafil for the Treatment of Erectile Dysfunction at 24 and 36 Hours After Dosing: A Randomized Controlled Trial," *Urology* 62, no. 1 (2003): 121–25; F. Montorsi et al., "Vardenafil Provides Reliable Efficacy Over Time in Men with Erectile Dysfunction," *Urology* 64, no. 6 (2004): 1187–95; A. Morgentaler et al., "Efficacy and Safety of Tadalafil Across Ethnic Groups and Various Risk Factors in Men with Erectile Dysfunction: Use of a Novel Noninferiority Study Design," *Journal of Sexual Medicine* 3, no. 3 (May 2006): 492–503.

126 A few years ago Cialis: S. E. Althof et al., "Impact of Tadalafil Once Daily in Men with Erectile Dysfunction—Including a Report of the Partners' Evaluation," *Urology* 75, no. 6 (June 2010): 1358–63.

132 Most people assume: I. Goldstein et al., "Oral Sildenafil in the Treatment of Erectile Dysfunction," *New England Journal of Medicine* 338, no. 20 (May 1998): 1397–404.

133 However, as physicians gained experience: A. Morgentaler, "Clinical Crossroads: A 66-Year-Old Man with Sexual Dysfunction," *Journal of the American Medical Association* 291 (2004): 2994–3003.

8. A HUSBAND'S DUTY

138 Jose was right: J. Rajfer, A. Rosciszewski, and M. Mehringer, "Prevalence of Corporeal Venous Leakage in Impotent Men," *Journal of Urology* 140, no. 1 (July 1988): 69–71.

143 Jose arrived in a special: J. J. Bookstein et al., "Penile Pharmacocavernosography and Cavernosometry in the Evaluation of Impotence," *Journal of Urology* 137, no. 4 (April 1987): 772–76.

146 Jose did well for six months: D. Schultheiss et al., "Long-term Results Following Dorsal Penile Vein Ligation in 126 Patients with Veno-Occlusive Dysfunction," *International Journal of Impotence Research* 9, no. 4 (December 1997): 205–9.

147 The problem for men with nerve injuries like Duncan's: J. J. Wyndaele et al., "Intracavernous Injection of Vasoactive Drugs, an Alternative for Treating Impotence in Spinal Cord Injury Patients," *Paraplegia* 24, no. 5 (October 1986): 271–75.

9. THE BIONIC PENIS

152 Early surgical ideas: C. E. Friley Jr., "Preparation and Preservation of the Baculum of Mammals," *Journal of Mammology* 28, no. 4 (November 1947): 395–97; "Baculum," Wikipedia entry (http://en.wikipedia.org/wiki/Baculum), accessed October 25, 2012.

153 The big conceptual advance: S. Lazarou, L. Reyes-Vallejo, and A. Morgentaler, "Technical Advances in Penile Prostheses," *Journal of Long-Term Effects of Medical Implants* 16, no. 3 (2006): 235–47; M. Lux et al., "Outcomes and Satisfaction Rates for the Redesigned 2-Piece Penile Prosthesis," *Journal of Urology* 177, no. 1 (January 2007): 262–66.

157 The implants are often considered: A. T. Guay et al., "Clinical Experience with Intraurethral Alprostadil (MUSE) in the Treatment of Men with Erectile Dysfunction: A Retrospective Study," *European Urology* 38, no. 6 (December 2000): 671–76.

165 Vincent did well with his surgery: H. J. Ramsawh et. al., "Quality of Life Following Simultaneous Placement of Penile Prosthesis with Radical Prostatectomy," *Journal of Urology* 174, no. 4 (October 2005): 1395–98.

10. MALE MENOPAUSE

174 One of the fastest-growing: A. Morgentaler, *Testosterone for Life: Recharge Your Vitality, Sex Drive, Muscle Mass and Overall Health* (New York: McGraw-Hill, 2009).

175 "Dr. Morgentaler, I read about you": S. Somers, *Bombshell: Explosive Medical Secrets That Will Redefine Aging* (New York: Crown Archetype, 2012).

180 William lay down on his left side: W. Conners, K. Flinn, and A.Morgentaler, "Outcomes with the 'V' Implantation Technique vs. Standard Technique for Testosterone Pellet Therapy," *Journal of Sexual Medicine*, online publication, December 8, 2011; A. R. McCullough et al., "A Multi-Institutional Observational Study of

Testosterone Levels after Testosterone Pellet (Testopel®) Insertion," *Journal of Sexual Medicine*, online publication, January 12, 2012.

184 The experiment was a home run: A. Morgentaler and D. Crews, "Role of the Anterior Hypothalamus-Preoptic Area in the Regulation of Reproductive Behavior in the Lizard, *Anolis carolinensis*: Implantation Studies," *Hormones and Behavior* 11 (1978): 61.

187 Testosterone acts on the brains: A. M. Traish et al., "Adipocyte Accumulation in Penile Corpus Cavernosum of the Orchiectomized Rabbit: A Potential Mechanism for Veno-occlusive Dysfunction in Androgen Deficiency," *Journal of Andrology* 26, no. 2 (March/April 2005): 242–48.

187 In another rabbit experiment: A. M. Traish et al., "Effects of Castration and Androgen Replacement on Erectile Function in a Rabbit Model," *Endocrinology* 140, no. 4 (April 1999): 1861–68.

188 If a man comes to see me: A. Morgentaler, "Clinical Crossroads: A 66-Year-Old Man with Sexual Dysfunction," *Journal of the American Medical Association* 291 (2004): 2994–3003; L. Reyes-Vallejo, S. Lazarou, and A. Morgentaler, "Subjective Sexual Response to Testosterone Replacement Therapy Based on Initial Serum Levels of Total Testosterone," *Journal of Sexual Medicine* 4 (2007): 1757–62.

188 Researchers in Taiwan: T. I. Hwang et al., "Combined Use of Androgen and Sildenafil for Hypogonadal Patients Unresponsive to Sildenafil Alone," *International Journal of Impotence Research* 18, no. 4 (July/August 2006): 400–404.

192 For the last twenty years: C. Huggins, and C. V. Hodges. "Studies on Prostatic Cancer: I. The Effect of Castration, of Estrogen and of Androgen Injection on Serum Phosphatases in Metastatic Carcinoma of the Prostate," *Cancer Research* 1 (1941): 293–97.

193 In the early 1990s I began: A. Morgentaler, C. O. Bruning III, and W. C. DeWolf, "Incidence of Occult Prostate Cancer Among Men with Low Total or Free Serum Testosterone," *Journal of the American Medical Association* 276 (1996): 1904–6.

193 Yet for a time: E. L. Rhoden and A. Morgentaler, "Risks of Testosterone-Replacement Therapy and Recommendations for Monitoring," *New England Journal of Medicine* 350 (2004): 482–92; A. Morgentaler, "Testosterone Replacement Therapy and Prostate Risks: Where's the Beef?" *Canadian Journal of Urology* 13 (2006): S40–43.

194 I found the volume: A. Morgentaler, "Testosterone and Prostate Cancer: An Historical Perspective on a Modern Myth," *European Urology* 50 (2006): 935–39.

194 It turns out that prostate: A. Morgentaler and A. Traish, "Shifting the Paradigm of Testosterone and Prostate Cancer: the Saturation Model and the Limits of Androgen-Dependent Growth," *European Urology* 55 (2009): 310–20.

194 In May 2011: A. Morgentaler et al., "Testosterone Therapy in Men with Untreated Prostate Cancer," *Journal of Urology* 185 (2011): 1256–61.

II. AM I NORMAL?

205 The male obsession with size: R. Shamloul, "Treatment of Men Complaining of Short Penis," *Urology* 65 (2005): 1183–85.

206 A common problem for men: J. Lever, D. A. Frederick, and L.A. Peplau, "Does Size Matter? Men's and Women's Views on Penis Size Across the Lifespan," *Psychology of Men and Masculinity* 7 (2006): 129–43; H. Ghanem et al., "Position Paper: Management of Men Complaining of a Small Penis Despite an Actually Normal Size," *Journal of Sexual Medicine*, online publication, April 18, 2012.

214 So, what is a normal penis size?: H. Wessels, T. F. Lue, and J. W. McAninch, "Penile Length in the Flaccid and Erect State: Guidelines for Penile Augmentation," *Journal of Urology* 156 (1996): 995–97.

217 The frequency with which we have sex: A. Nicolosi et al., "Sexual Behavior and Sexual Dysfunctions after Age 40: The Global Study of Sexual Attitudes and Behaviors," *Urology* 64, no. 5 (November 2004): 991–97; S. T. Lindau et al., "A Study of Sexuality and Health Among Older Adults in the United States," *New England Journal of Medicine* 357, no. 8 (August 2007): 762–74.

I2. NO BALLS AT ALL

236 Together with the resident: J. Maranchie and A. Morgentaler, "Management of Impending Sterility," *Lancet* 347 (1996): 1344.

239 A few years ago: C. P. Wu and F. L. Gu, "The Prostate in Eunuchs," *Progress in Clinical and Biological Research* 370 (1991): 249–55.

241 On June 1, 1889: C. E. Brown-Séquard, "The Effects Produced on Man by Subcutaneous Injections of a Liquid Obtained from the Testicles of Animals," *Lancet* 2 (1889): 105–7.

242 Eugen Steinach: E. Steinach, *Sex and Life: Forty Years of Biological and Medical Experiments* (London: Faber and Faber, 1940).

242 Serge Voronoff, a Russian émigré: N. L. Miller and B. R. Fulmer, "Injection, Ligation and Transplantation: The Search for the Glandular Fountain of Youth," *Journal of Urology* 177 (2007): 2000–2005.

13. NARCISSUS AND THE PENIS REFLECTED

246 The prevalence of homosexuality: M. Diamond, "Homosexuality and Bisexuality in Different Populations," *Archives of Sexual Behavior* 22, no. 4 (August 1993): 291–310; A. C. Kinsey, W. B. Pomeroy, and C. E. Martin, *Sexual Behavior in the Human Male* (Bloomington: Indiana University Press, 1975; first published 1948); E. O. Laumann et al., *The Social Organization of Sexuality: Sexual Practices in the United States* (Chicago: University of Chicago Press, 1994); R. L. Sell, J. A. Wells, and D. D. Wypij, "The Prevalence of Homosexual Behavior and Attraction in the United States, the United Kingdom and France: Results of National Population-Based Samples," *Archives of Sexual Behavior* 24, no. 3 (1995): 235–48; T. Joloza et al., "Measuring Sexual Identity: Evaluation Report, 2010," Office for National Statistics (UK), September 23, 2010, www.ons.gov.uk/ons/rel/ethnicity/measur ing-sexual-identity—evaluation-report/2010/index.html, accessed online October 25, 2012; D. M. Smith and G. J. Gates, "Gay and Lesbian Families in the United States: Same-Sex Unmarried Partner House- holds: A Preliminary Analysis of 2000 United States Census Data: A Human Rights Campaign Report," Urban Institute, August 22, 2001, http://www.urban.org/UploadedPDF/1000491_gl_partner_house holds.pdf, accessed October 25, 2012.

249 One of the great mysteries: V. Puppo and I. Gruenwald, "Does the G-spot Exist? A Review of the Current Literature," *International Urogynecology Journal*, published online, June 6, 2012.

14. MEN ARE PEOPLE TOO!

264 It is difficult to be a man these days: "For Women Under 30, Most Births Occur Outside Marriage," *New York Times*, February 17, 2012; Hannah Rosin, "The End of Men," *Atlantic*, July/August 2010.

267 A poorly recognized additional challenge: H. A. Feldman et al., "Impotence and Its Medical and Psychosocial Correlates: Results of the Massachusetts Male Aging Study," *Journal of Urology* 151, no. 1 (1994): 54–61.

267 Declining levels of testosterone: T. Mulligan et al., "Prevalence of Hypogonadism in Males Aged at Least 45 Years: The HIM Study," *International Journal of Clinical Practice* 60, no. 7 (July 2006): 762–69.

268 the futurist Raymond Kurzweil: R. Kurzweil, *The Singularity Is Near* (New York: Penguin Books, 2006).

castration. Removal of the testicles.

castrato (singular), **castrati** (plural). Male singers who underwent surgical treatment to prevent puberty—and thus deepening of their voices—by castration or by injuring the blood supply to the testicles.

clitoris. The sensitive button of tissue above the vagina that is the female anatomic equivalent of the penis.

climax. Synonymous with orgasm.

corona. The crown, or ridge, that forms the part of the head of the penis that is closest to the body.

corpus cavernosum (singular), **corpora cavernosa** (plural). The two paired chambers of the penis responsible for erection.

corpus spongiosum: The structure that runs along the underside of the penis, containing the urethra. Toward the tip of the penis the corpus spongiosum flares out to become the glans.

dewlap. Lax skin under the jaw. In male lizards the dewlap is brightly colored and is extended and displayed during sexual behaviors.

ejaculation. The expulsion of seminal fluid.

emasculation. Removal of testicles and penis.

erectile dysfunction (ED). Reduced ability to achieve or maintain adequate erections for intercourse.

exstrophy. A congenital condition in which the bladder appears on the exterior of the abdominal wall at birth, often associated with genital and urethral abnormalities.

glans. The head of the penis.

gonad. Ovary or testicle.

hermaphrodite. An individual with male and female gonads, namely testis and ovary.

hypospadias. A congenital condition in which the urethral tube formation is incomplete, resulting in an opening somewhere along the underside of the shaft or head of the penis.

hypothalamus. A deep portion of the brain responsible for several key biological functions, including regulation of the pituitary gland to help maintain normal testosterone levels.

impotence. Erectile dysfunction. The term is now largely abandoned in the United States, but still in use elsewhere in the world.

in vitro fertilization (IVF). Process to achieve pregnancy in which sperm from the man and eggs from the woman are combined in a laboratory dish. Once fertilized, one or more eggs are then placed in the woman's uterus so that a pregnancy can then occur.

karyotype. Genetic test to determine the number and integrity of chromosomes. A normal male karyotype is 46XY, indicating a total of 46 chromosomes, including a Y and an X chromosome. A normal female karyotype is 46XX.

labia. The folds of skin on the exterior of a woman's genital region, surrounding the opening to the vagina.

Müllerian ducts. Primitive fetal structures that are destined to form the female reproductive structures—Fallopian tubes, uterus, and upper two-thirds of vagina.

neonatal. The time period soon after birth.

orgasm. The physical and psychological experiences at the peak of the sexual experience, generally followed by a sense of release.

phallus. Penis or clitoris. Some authorities, particularly British, restrict this term only to the erect structure.

pituitary. A hormone-producing part of the brain.

prostate. Walnut-sized gland in the male pelvis that sits at the opening of the bladder. The prostate produces approximately one-third of the seminal fluid during ejaculation.

pseudohermaphrodite. An individual with some combination of apparent male and female genital structures, but only one type of gonad—either testis or ovary.

testicular torsion. A twist of the testicles on their blood supply, usually leading to necrosis (death) of the testicle if untreated.

testosterone. A hormone produced primarily by the testicles in men (smaller amounts are also produced in men and women by the adrenals).

tunica albuginea. Tough sheath that surrounds the corpora cavernosa of the penis. Also the name of the tough membrane that forms the surface of the testicles.

urethra. The tube that runs from the bladder to the outside. In men this tube carries urine and semen. In women it carries only urine.

vas deferens (singular), **vasa deferentia** (plural). The tube that normally carries sperm and testicular fluid that runs from the epididymis to the prostate, where it joins with the duct from the seminal vesicles.

vasectomy. Procedure in which the vas deferens is cut and tied off. Used as a permanent form of male contraception.

vasectomy reversal. Procedure to reconnect the ends of the vas deferens that were divided during vasectomy, usually performed to reestablish fertility.

veno-occlusive dysfunction. Impaired trapping of blood within the corpora cavernosa during erection, leading to ED.

venous ligation. An operation to treat veno-occlusive dysfunction by tying off (ligating) the veins draining the penis.

Wolffian ducts. Primitive fetal structures that are destined to form several of the male reproductive structures—the vas deferens, seminal vesicles, and epididymis.

ADDITIONAL READING

Friedman, David M. *A Mind of Its Own: A Cultural History of the Penis*. New York: Free Press, 2001.

Kinsey, A. C., W. B. Pomeroy, and C. E. Martin. *Sexual Behavior in the Human Male*. Bloomington: Indiana University Press, 1975 (first published in 1948).

Masters, William H., and Virginia E. Johnson. *Human Sexual Inadequacy*. Boston: Little, Brown, 1970.

Morgentaler, Abraham. *The Male Body: A Physician's Guide to What Every Man Should Know about His Sexual Health*. New York: Fireside/Simon and Schuster, 1993.

———. *The Viagra Myth: The Surprising Impact on Love and Relationships*. San Francisco: Jossey Bass/Wiley, 2003.

———. *Testosterone for Life: Recharge Your Vitality, Sex Drive, Muscle Mass and Overall Health*. New York: McGraw-Hill, 2009.

Roach, Mary. *Bonk: The Curious Coupling of Science and Sex*. New York: W. W. Norton, 2008.

ACKNOWLEDGMENTS

This book is the result of my good fortune in having come to know several of the most dynamic people on this planet. The delightful Anita Waxman got me started with her introduction into the inner circle of publishing. Bob Levine, agent extraordinaire, trusted advisor, and, ultimately, my unofficial senior editor, worked with me from initial concept through the final draft. I could not have written this book without his wisdom and guidance. My publisher, the remarkably accomplished Steve Rubin, took a chance on an unknown author with an unusual book idea and invested his own considerable energy and insight to give this project a fighting chance for success. I am grateful for his vision and encouragement.

I'd like to thank my team at Holt, particularly my editors Marjorie Braman and Joanna Levine, who made me sound more articulate than I am. I wish to thank Mark Greenberg, Laurence Glickman, MD, and Ken Lester, lifelong friends who provided valuable feedback on various chapters. A special thank-you to the oh-so-wise Cindy Whitehead, who read every word of the manuscript, encouraged me to write what I thought was true, and kept me focused on the big picture. A big hug and a kiss for the tops of their heads to my wonderful daughters, Maya and Hannah, who remind me every day what is most important in life. I am blessed as well to have had the support of my sister, Dr. Goldie Morgentaler, and her husband, Dr. Jonathan Seldin; my brother Yann and his wife, Melyssa; my brother Ben Morgentaler; and my stepmother Arlene Leibovitch.

We are each the products of our histories and our inspirations. Ma, I think of you every day and miss you terribly. Ta, you've been the best father a man could ever have. What a world of possibility the two of you have given me!

For the past thirteen years my staff at Men's Health Boston has provided a unique experience for men and their partners—friendly, professional, reassuring—that has given me the opportunity to explore a world with my patients that requires trust and confidence. I could not do what I do without them.

Finally, and most importantly, I must thank my patients for having the courage to share with me their stories of intimacy. Doing so has provided me with a window into the subtleties of human experience. The men and women who have graced me with their honesty have been my teachers: whatever kernels of wisdom are contained in this book come directly from them.

Index

ABOUT THE AUTHOR

DR. ABRAHAM MORGENTALER is an associate clinical professor of urology at Harvard Medical School and the founder and director of Men's Health Boston, the first comprehensive center in the United States devoted to the specialized medical needs of men. He is the author of three previous books, *Testosterone for Life*, *The Viagra Myth*, and *The Male Body* and his pioneering work in the fields of male sexuality, testosterone deficiency, and prostate cancer has appeared in medical journals such as *The New England Journal of Medicine* and *The Lancet*, as well as in popular media including *The New Yorker* and *The Wall Street Journal*. Dr. Morgentaler lectures internationally, conducts research, and continues to see patients. He lives and works near Boston.